My Physical Scars are *Beautiful:*

They Represent God's Answer to Prayer

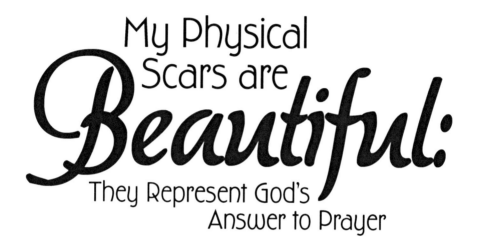

Sandy Blank

WestBow
PRESS
A DIVISION OF THOMAS NELSON

WestBow Press books may be ordered through booksellers or by contacting:

WestBow Press
A Division of Thomas Nelson
1663 Liberty Drive
Bloomington, IN 47403
www.westbowpress.com
1-(866) 928-1240

Because of the dynamic nature of the Internet, any web addresses or links contained in this book may have changed since publication and may no longer be valid. The views expressed in this work are solely those of the author and do not necessarily reflect the views of the publisher, and the publisher hereby disclaims any responsibility for them.

Any people depicted in stock imagery provided by Thinkstock are models, and such images are being used for illustrative purposes only.

Certain stock imagery © Thinkstock.

ISBN: 978-1-4497-7433-2 (sc)
ISBN: 978-1-4497-7434-9 (hc)
ISBN: 978-1-4497-7432-5 (e)

Library of Congress Control Number: 2012921200

Printed in the United States of America

WestBow Press rev. date: 11/13/2012

Preface

I picked up a daily devotional book the other day and the reading was, "_Tell Your Story_". I thought, _Was God trying to tell me something?_ I didn't think my story would be any different than anyone else's story that had been severely injured in a vehicle or a motorcycle accident. I prayed others would find similarities and comfort in my book, if I were to write one. I thought, if I were to share my experiences and struggles, others would be able to relate—to understand God has a purpose and a time for everything. Even the awful things that happen in our lives can be used for good.

I have never been a writer; but, I have felt compelled, by God, to write this book. I felt everyone who read my book would see how His plans have worked in my life and in my family's lives. Some of what I have told you will be hard to believe, even harder to understand. From my perspective everything is true. Remember, I was pretty heavily medicated, especially in the beginning. However, I do have all of the haunting memories of things that went on around me, medicated or not. At times, I felt God and His Angels were all I had; even though I was surrounded by doctors, nurses, aides, housekeepers, church family, and my personal family. I felt alone with my thoughts and God.

Acknowledgements

I wish to thank so many people; I don't know where to begin. Over the last six years, each and every person has contributed something to my life. People whose names I never knew, can't remember, or have changed for the purpose of writing this book. And, I keep running into people out of the clear blue-- who add bits and pieces to my story. That has been a beautiful thing.

My main doctor, Dr. Nabil Ebraheim, Orthopedic Doctor at TU Medical Center (Dr. Nabil Ebraheim, Personal Communication, August 11, 2011) was the doctor I was delivered to via helicopter. Probably a month into my situation, amputation of my left leg was still being considered. I asked the doctor if he was going to take my leg off, and he responded, "I'm a fighter". His comment was all I needed to hear. The *fight* was on! Thank you from the bottom of my heart for being "a fighter". After my book is published, I will bring you a copy.

I want to thank the crew of the Life-Flite helicopter that transported me to the hospital. A special thank you to the nurse on board, whose name I don't know; but, is responsible for diverting the helicopter to the best hospital and the best doctor for my injuries. I owe many thanks to all the hospital staff, as well. They worked extremely hard keeping me alive and putting the pieces back together. I was like *'Humpty Dumpty'* when I first arrived. I was told by an x-ray tech that I was one patient the staff was watching with considerable interest from May 2006 up to and including today. Many times I heard the word **miracle.**

I want to thank my husband, Wayne, for hanging around the last six years, and being there for me through all my ups and downs; and, believe me, there were many! It was a long haul and certainly was not easy. Wayne was at my bedside every day and waited, alone, though every operation. Over a four year period, I was either in the hospital or a nursing home; and, Wayne was busy volunteering. He got involved in politics, the NRA, Vets, Inc., AM Vets, American Legion, and the American Legion Riders. "I love you".

I love my daughter, Aprell, and granddaughter, Brandi. They were at the accident scene; which was terribly traumatic for them. My youngest granddaughter, Brittany, I love you too. She was not at the accident scene nor was she allowed to visit me for a couple of months due to the nature of my injuries. *Thank you* all for your support, love, and the picture of my cat, Tigger. That picture hung on the walls and accompanied me to every nursing home.

My church was incredible. The congregation pulled together for us: the visits, cards, flowers, support, encouragement, dinners, and most of all the prayers. The many prayers were appreciated and will never be forgotten. I contribute the Prayers as to why I am still on this earth; and, God's plan. *Thank you.*

My co-workers at the Probation/Parole Department in Monroe, MI were immensely supportive too. The Chief District Court Probation Officer drew up two get well posters for me. He asked many people at the Courthouse to sign each poster with their well wishes, and, mailed them to me. I hung the posters on the walls of the nursing homes. They were encouraging reminders that many people were thinking and praying for my recovery. *Thank you.*

In Christ,

Sandra L. Blank

Contents

Chapter I

Sunday, May 28, 2006—is a date engraved in my memory forever. My husband and I got up and went to Bible class, our usual Sunday morning ritual. After Sunday school, we went to lunch and then home, which was also our normal routine. On this particular day, though, we had time before the 6:00 p.m. service to go for a motorcycle ride. The day was sunny, hot, and beautiful without a cloud in the sky. It was a fantastic day for a ride. Wayne wanted to make one stop while we were out and about. I didn't care. I was excited!

I was riding my own bike, a Yamaha 1100, all decked out with lots of chrome; it was a sparkly dark brown, so dark it looked black. I felt pretty footloose and fancy-free, even though I followed Wayne on every ride. I never knew for sure where he wanted to go, so he led and I followed—no controversy that way. On our way through town, a couple of our friends, who were sitting in a little coffee shop on the corner, saw us ride by. We stopped at a political call center (it was an election year) to help clean it so it could be opened. It was so hot! I couldn't wait to get on the road! We were not dressed for being inside. It was just too hot! The wind from the motorcycle ride would cool us off some.

Finally, Wayne said we should go. Upon leaving the call center, Wayne suggested we ride to Ida, MI and get an ice cream. I was all for that! The ice-cream parlor was extremely busy, which was no wonder because it was so hot! After we parked and went inside, we waited awhile before we got our order, and then we had to stand to eat it. I spotted a young lady I knew from the courthouse, so we ate and talked. It was turning out to be a pleasant day. Then it was time to head for church. The ice cream had hit the spot, and I was a happy camper!

We started our bikes, left the parking lot, and turned south on Lewis Avenue and then right onto Albain Road—a back road that was bumpy and arched high in the middle with potholes or filled holes on the berm. We came upon a curve, and I slowed down, as I always do. Vehicles don't always slow for curves, though, especially on those back roads, so I checked my rearview mirror and saw what appeared to be a pickup truck behind me. He seemed to be following rather closely, and we all know "Objects in the mirrors *are* closer than they appear." I was hoping he would slow down when I did. Up ahead of me, Wayne was already into the curve. I will never forget the image of his back and his black leather vest.

What ... what's happening? I heard voices in my head! *I don't see anything... What's going on?* I was peering at a blank canvas. There wasn't anything—just blackness. I couldn't see anything, but I heard voices. I felt as if I was "out-of-body" or something. The voices were talking about how this was a good place for an accident. *An accident!?* The voice from my left told me, *Go right off the road!* I thought, *No! No! Not good! Not good at all!* However, I wasn't included in the conversation. I was on the outside looking in-not in control. My head seemed to be in between the two voices.

I couldn't see anything, but I could hear what was being argued about. I felt like there was a little person on my left shoulder, encouraging an accident, and another little person on my right shoulder, desperately trying to stop such a thing—like in the cartoons, where the little devil is on the left and the little angel is on the right. *Only, this is not funny! This is not a cartoon! This is happening! And it's happening to* me! I wasn't in control. Something was definitely not right.

I could still hear the voices, arguing back and forth. Then, all of a sudden, I was awake and was looking down at my bike. *What the ...? The bike is wobbling badly! What's going on? How do I stop it? Someone tell me what to do!* And then—*poof*—I was out of it again. I was there physically, but mentally, I felt as if I was in a trance or something. I didn't pass out, as some think. I didn't feel faint or sick to my stomach, nor was I sweating from the heat. In my head, I heard the voice on my right say, "No! Sandy! No! Don't! Oh—*sigh- -too late.*" That was it--nothing else. It was as if someone turned the lights out--complete darkness.

I don't remember hearing anything, seeing anything, or feeling anything. It was as if I were in a deep sleep. You know the kind: you go to sleep and the next thing you know, you're awake—nothing in between. I don't have a clue what went on after the lights went out or even how much time actually passed. It seemed time stood still.

A couple years later, I talked to a lady at church who had basically the same experience when she had her car accident. The people inside the first car she hit said she came at them like she was in a trance. She didn't see them; she just dropped her head to her chest and hit them. That is exactly what witnesses said about me—that I dropped my head to my chest and hit the vehicle. I didn't see the vehicle coming at me. I didn't panic, I wasn't sleepy, I wasn't nauseated, I felt no fear, nor did I feel pain. I believe God had a plan that day and He let Satan take control.

Later, I heard Wayne yelling, "Save her! Save her! Do whatever it takes! Save her!" I thought *He does love me. But what happened? What's going on? Where am I? Why did Wayne say that?* I thought I was lying down and then I was being carried. On my left, I thought there was a figure next to my head. In my mind, Wayne was somewhere near the top of my head, slowly running toward me, like in the movies when two people run toward each other in slow motion. Then he stopped. The visions in my head were of hospital-like surroundings, and I heard nurses talking. Again, I felt like I was physically there, but I couldn't talk or move. I thought I was lying quiet, but for how long, I don't remember.

When I came to later, I had the impression that I was in a wheelchair and that Wayne was pushing me. He stopped; someone was talking to him. I couldn't believe how groggy I felt. I looked up at what appeared to be an elevator door. It was cold, and the walls were gray, institutional or hospital looking. I heard a woman's voice tell me, "Wait. I'll be right with you," and I nodded. I heard other voices too, but I don't know what was said. The elevator opened, and I was pushed into a small metallic room. Then the lights went out again.

At that point, I was not totally conscious; but, I believe, I walked (staggered was more like it) around inside a big building. I could hear people all around me, but no one was paying any attention to the fact that I was not steady on my feet and looked terribly lost. I wandered between partitions, curtains, chairs, and tables or beds. Finally, a lady told me to sit or lie down. When she asked me my name, I told her, "Sandy." She told me to wait a minute and she would be back.

I wondered where Wayne had gone. I didn't see anyone I knew; even the surroundings were unfamiliar. I guessed I would sit for a minute on the table, behind a curtain; then, a few minutes later, I had to lie down. The lady came back to check on me and then left again. There was so much confusion in my head.

Wait! I think I hear familiar voices. Can't be, can it? A woman I worked with, a probation officer. I struggled to get up far enough to peek through the curtain. I wanted to make sure the people talking were the people I thought they were. *It is! What's going on?* I didn't want them to see me for some reason. I thought she was having a conversation with a man. I peeked through the curtain again. It was her husband, a police officer. They were talking about using their daughter as a decoy in a sting operation of some kind. *They can't do that! Their daughter is beautiful. She's only nineteen, tall with long, naturally curly brown hair. She'll get hurt.* I peeked through the curtain again. I could see their daughter in my mind, standing there with her long hair hanging down her back, wearing a waist-length, light-colored jacket, a very short black skirt, and very high red heels. I thought we were in an airport. I was so tired and had to lie back down. I listened for a while to the voices on the other side of the curtain and heard the operation the police officer and probation officer were planning, which sounded like some kind of a drug bust in the making. *Can this be right?*

Morphine allows a person to concoct all sorts of scenarios in their minds. Some of the people I worked with were in my mind, thoughts and dreams.

The lady came back and gave me what I thought was a shot in my right arm. I didn't know what was going on. Someone else I thought was wrapping my left arm, and, someone else was talking to me on the other side-I didn't know who anyone was. I felt so mixed up and confused!

Wayne was there. He came around a partition, and walked up to me. He was talking, but, I couldn't connect with him. I thought he asked me what I was doing. He told me I needed to lay still. Around the same partition came the lady from earlier. She brought a young man with her dressed in nursing clothes (scrubs); dark blue shirt and pants with a stethoscope around his neck. This young man was tall, slim, with dark brown wavy hair, a big smile, and his teeth were real white. He came over to us and asked me how I felt. He told Wayne he was taking me somewhere--I couldn't make out where he said. My movements were slow and sluggish. I couldn't quite get it all together for some reason. I asked the young man if he was an ambulance driver, and he responded that he was going to drive me someplace. Then Wayne left. *Where did he go?* The young man said Wayne would return later and he pushed me, on a gurney, to a waiting vehicle. I could not see any markings on the vehicle; but, Wayne was inside and so were other people—I didn't know any of them. We were driving to an unknown place—I didn't know where. The young man said we needed to stop for gas and some people needed to eat. He pulled the vehicle into a gas station, at least, that's what I thought it was. It was getting late and the sun was going down. Wayne and the others got out of the vehicle and went inside the gas station for food and drink. In my head, I slowly got out of the vehicle and walked around with a soft cast on my left leg and crutches. I stumbled and someone told me to be careful. I responded, "I'm alright".

I got into what I thought was a glass sided elevator and it broke down with me inside. I was very scared! I couldn't move! I looked down and the floor was gone! I stood on the ledge, which was about four inches wide. In my mind, I could not see a floor. The young man walked over to the elevator and began to encourage me. He asked me to go to an open window on the other side of the elevator and get out. He reached in the elevator with his hand leaning in toward me. *I just can't do it! I'm going to fall if I do. There's no bottom.* I froze! The young man--talked to me trying to calm me. We talked for… what seemed a long while. Then, he said he had to leave his family was waiting for him; but, he would be back tomorrow. He told me Wayne had to go home too.

A few minutes later—what appeared to me to be a State Police car pulled up outside the elevator. A short, stocky, younger lady with long blonde hair wearing a State Police uniform got out of the car and came over to us. The young man explained that the young lady would be staying with me while he and Wayne were gone. They talked for a minute ut of ear shot of me and then he left. The young lady was a very nice understanding person--soft spoken. She also attempted to talk me out of the elevator. I didn't cooperate. She tried to get into the elevator through the window to help get me out--she couldn't get in. There were too many things on her belt that kept getting caught on the sides of the window and on the glass. A call came through on the car radio and the young lady left. I didn't like her leaving me alone. I felt as if I was in an interrogation room--there was a light shining down on me. It was very dark outside. I could see my reflection in the windows and nothing outside. I didn't know how many times Linda came back; I knew it was a lot. She asked me if I wanted her to call Wayne, and I nodded *yes,* however, it was too late at night. The young lady told me he would be there in the morning. I understood everything she told me. She left again and I went to sleep.

In my mind, I was still standing in this glass elevator on a very narrow ledge with no floor. I was anxious and felt very much alone. I took a step out, looked down, and fear gripped my chest. My heart started pumping real fast as if it were going to jump out of my chest. I pushed myself back up against the wall of the elevator and waited for help. The place was empty, there was no one around, and, like I said, it was very dark outside of the elevator. I prayed, *Lord, help me be patient.* I slipped off to sleep. I don't remember anything else.

I just described my perception of the motorcycle accident as it happened in my mind. The rest of the book is the next five years; as I remembered them or as the events were relayed to me by other people.

Chapter II

It was Memorial Day, May 28, 2006, about 5:15 p.m.---a very nice evening. It was *hot*, but a good evening for a ride. We had just eaten ice cream at the ice cream parlor and were heading for church. The crash was heard all over the neighborhood and people came running from everywhere. My brother-in-law's step-daughter was at a house party nearby. She came running to the scene as fast as she could. Her lady friend a nurse was at the same house party; she also came running to the scene as fast as she could. The accident vehicles stopped in the nurse's driveway--right in front of her house. The nurse's husband witnessed the accident. He was outside in his yard when the sound of the motorcycles caught his attention. He turned around in time to see me collide with a Jeep Cherokee. He said he thought I flew through the air about thirty feet and landed in the roadway near my bike. The Jeep continued to skid in a half circle, collided with the trailer the pickup following me was pulling, and knocked the Jet Ski off the trailer.

My husband saw me, in his review mirror, impact the vehicle; he did not see how the accident happened. Wayne panicked, locking up the brakes on his bike, trying to stop and get back to me. Luckily he did not dump his bike too. The man at the house called his wife on her cell phone, but, she was already on her way to the scene. She and my step-niece were running like two kids down the road. My niece sat down in the road putting my head between her legs to keep me quiet and immobile. I had woken up, was talking, and wanted to stand up. The nurse got on her cell phone and called for Life-Flite. She didn't have the authority to summon the helicopter to the accident scene; but, she tried to convey that I would die unless they came. The ambulance was on its way. It was just not quick enough. It was determined; I would not have made it in the ambulance. The hospital was too far away and the road too bumpy. The nurse was afraid I was going into shock. She got so upset with all the people standing around not doing anything; but, she and my niece were the only two medical people on the scene. They were only qualified to treat me for shock, take my vitals and call for help. My injuries were extensive and they were limited in what they could do.

Back at the house party, a friend of ours from church and her family and friends formed a circle, held hands, and began praying for the accident victim. At the time they were unaware of who the victim was. Her husband came out to the scene, saw that it was Wayne and me and went back to the house to tell his wife. She immediately called the telephone prayer line at church and started people praying for me. Knowing who the accident victim was only intensified our friends' prayers and the urgency to get the word of my accident out to the other members of our church.

To Wayne it seemed an eternity for the fire department to finally arrive at the scene; and, by that time he was a real basket case. The sight of so much blood and all my broken bones hanging out everywhere was more than he could handle.

My brother-in-law heard about the accident over his police scanner. He called my daughter, Aprell, and granddaughter, Brandi. They all arrived at the accident scene about the same time. Brandi began running to me and was commandeered by a police officer before she could reach me. She and Wayne were extremely upset and fire department personnel put them in the ambulance in hopes they would calm down. Neither of them stayed in the ambulance though. Brandi was eventually put in the front seat of the ambulance, and the nurse attempted to put her mind at ease with conversation. At that point, I'm not sure where Aprell or Wayne was.

At some point my brother-in-law called the rest of the family. He relayed the news that the situation did not look good--not good at all. The fire chief, a friend and member of our church, called for the Life-Flite helicopter informing them that I couldn't be transported to the hospital in Monroe. He claimed an ambulance ride would certainly be the end of me. The Life Flite was already in route to someplace else but advised the Chief if he could have me ready to transport within ten minutes, they would divert to pick me up. He confirmed I would be ready and that there was a small field across from the scene they could land in.

The Life Flite nurse on board observed the severity of all my injuries and diverted the helicopter a second time to the Trauma Unit at a hospital in Toledo, Ohio. He knew of a very well-known orthopedic doctor at that hospital, so he determined I was in desperate need of that doctor. God's plan was definitely in the works and He was definitely in control.

The fire chief's son arrived on the scene looking for his Dad. They were supposed to have met someplace on business. When the Chief didn't show for their meeting, his son checked to see if he was on a call and came out to the scene. The Chief's son was a volunteer fireman also and he too belonged to the same church as Wayne and me. He arrived, just as things were wrapping up. Following his observation of what had taken place and who was involved, he drove back into town to our church—interrupting the service to tell our Pastor about the accident. Pastor announced the news of the accident, and my extremely grave condition. I have been told there were many, many prayers sent to God right then and there. The fire chief's son waited until after the service to transport our Pastor to the hospital.

The fire chief transported Wayne to the hospital from the scene, as Wayne was too upset to drive himself. Our friends from church took Wayne's motorcycle into their daughter's garage for safekeeping until he could return to pick it up. My brother-in-law went to the hospital along with my mother-in-law and sister-in-law. Prior to Aprell leaving for the hospital she stopped to talk to a police officer about the accident. The officer picked up my helmet from the ground, started to hand it to Aprell, then said, "I can't give you this, it's a fatal", and he put the helmet back down on the ground. Obviously, my daughter was overwhelmed with grief and ran to her car crying so hard she could barely see to drive.

Brandi and Aprell were all set to leave for Brandi's eighth grade class trip the next morning, May 29, 2006 at 8:00 a.m. They were suppose to go to Chicago, Illinois for four days. Aprell would not go on the class trip knowing I could die within the next few minutes or days. However, she wanted Brandi to go on her trip so she took her to one of her girlfriends prior to leaving for the hospital. The principal of Trinity School promised Aprell he would keep Brandi informed of all changes with me. A couple of the parents, who were driving to Chicago, promised to bring Brandi home as soon as possible if my condition worsened or I died; which, was a very good possibility at the time.

My injuries were life-threatening. I broke my right tibia (right leg), left tibia and fibula (left leg-both bones), left femur (thigh), left knee, left and right wrists, left ring and little fingers, left radius and ulna (lower arm-both bones), humerus (upper arm), and blew out my left elbow totally. All these breaks were compound---bones through the skin. I also cracked my pelvis and some ribs. I had internal bleeding; ruptured spleen, and severed my liver. My body turned black and blue and I swelled beyond recognition. The EMTS attendants made two slits on the tops of my left and right hands, one slit inside each finger of my left hand, and two slits on the top of my left foot--to relieve the pressure and keep my skin from splitting.

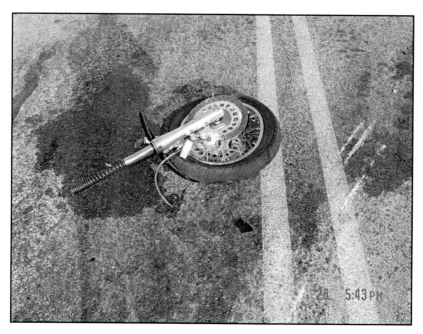

Motorcycle front wheel

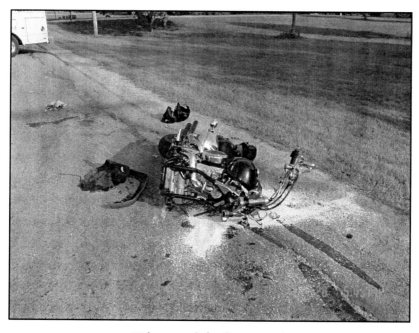

What was left of motorcycle

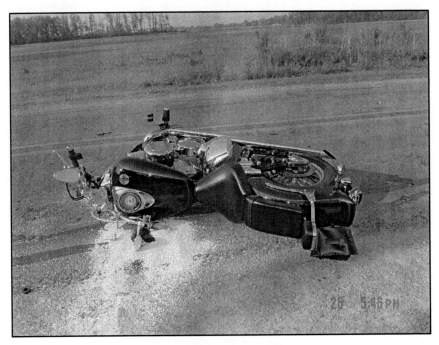

What was left of motorcycle

My arrival at the hospital trauma unit alive was a blessing in itself. I had been told they lost me once while in flight, but I was breathing when I arrived at the hospital—where personnel was waiting and went right to work. They began by sucking the blood and debris out of my wounds. They wanted to see the extent of the injuries because my abdomen felt as if there was fluid accumulating inside. I had lost a great deal of blood and was given a transfusion of eight pints. I believe a person only has ten pints of blood in their body to begin with. Anyway, they x-rayed me from top to bottom; which was also close call. I am highly allergic to the ionic dye used in CT scans and that was the x-ray they were about to do. At the last minute, my daughter remembered my allergy, ran through the hospital to radiology to stop the technicians before they gave me the dye. Close call! She advised me that the IV was hooked up to my arm and they were within seconds of releasing the dye into my veins when she entered the room in a panic. An allergic reaction to that dye would have definitely been detrimental to my survival. I believe this was God's work. For Aprell to have even remembered my ionic dye allergy at such a traumatic time, I believe was a miracle in itself. Sometime later on during my recovery I talked to an x-ray tech at the hospital, who remembered my coming into the trauma unit. She helped set me up for the CT scan. She picked up my left leg... and...she sighed...it was like *mush*. Following the x-rays, they immediately took me to surgery where my spleen was removed and they searched for further sources of internal bleeding.

My wounds were cleaned, wrapped, and I was put on hold until I stabilized. The doctors didn't set my breaks at that time. They cleaned the areas as thoroughly as they could, pinned my legs together with titanium bars, and wrapped them. Both arms were put in casts, plus I had been stitched down the center of my abdomen from just under the rib cage to the top of the pubic hair line.

The doctors didn't give my family one iota of hope that I would make it through the night. The trauma unit doctor came down the stairs many times during the night to update my husband and family on my condition. The reports from the doctors were not good.

Wayne was distressed and those waiting with him tried to be of help by acting as his advocate. However, that wasn't the right moment. Wayne was offended; and, did not appreciate what they were attempting to do for him. He made his feelings known quickly. In the process of letting others know his feelings, he hurt other's feelings. Wayne understood what people were trying to do for him; but, to jump in without asking him if he minded wasn't a good decision. The stress Wayne was under at the time was enormous.

Comments that Wayne acted "like he's nuts!" along with looks of disgust and anger toward Wayne surprised me. The situation was dire; and, what Wayne had just witnessed was traumatic—war like. People should have understood he probably was not in a stable state of mind at that time--no one would have been. I can't help but wonder what the reactions would have been had the shoes been on someone else. Anyway, all this drama seemed pretty insignificant to me since I was *fighting for my life*.

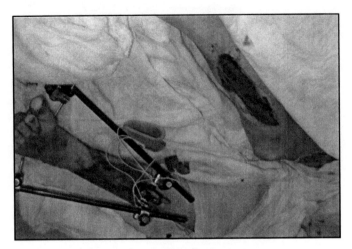

Rt & lt leg wounds

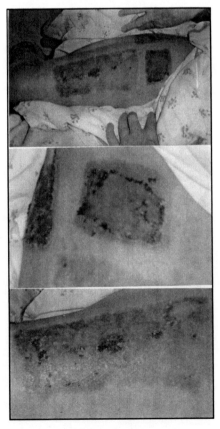

Lt. leg skin graphs

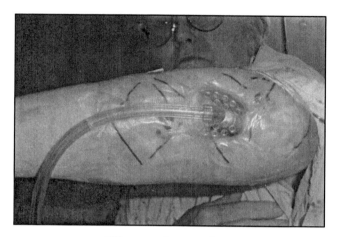

Elbow with wound vac

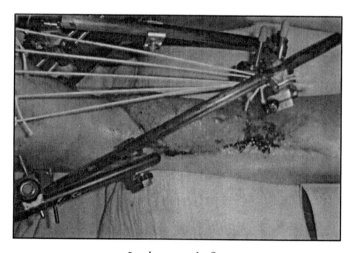

Lt. leg muscle flap

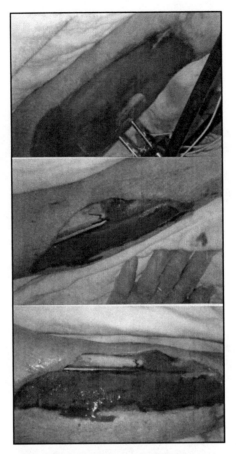

Left leg wound with plate showing

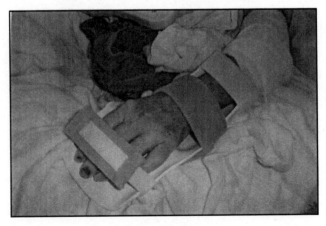

Lt. hand/elbow

The first night passed and I was still hanging in there: the second, third, fourth and fifth nights went by---I was still breathing. At some point, I was put in a medically induced coma for some three weeks.

I believe my accident happened for a reason. It was not *just* an accident. There was a reason. There was a purpose. There was a plan. It happened too perfectly. I mean the first people at the scene were family and friends from our church. The prayers were many and immediate. The volunteers from the fire department in attendance at the scene claimed, I am one in four to have survived such an accident. I totally believe God was in control of the whole situation. I do not remember anything about the vehicle coming toward me or the collision. There wasn't any fear, panic, or pain. In my opinion, the following explained to me, *why* my accident happened; a question I don't ever remember asking myself or anyone else. I believed, in my heart, I already knew the answer.

Chapter III

A Sunday in December 2005 or January 2006, my husband, Wayne, and I were in standing in the balcony of our church listening to our minister saying prayers for our congregation. For some reason this day the prayers were particularly concerning to me. Trinity was going through real troubling trials and I felt the prayers should have been more heartfelt or sincere. I don't know, more personal.

There was a script fund raiser started by our school from which $175,000.00 had been embezzled. No one knew where the monies went, who the guilty party was, or exactly who was responsible for monitoring the monies in the first place. Finger pointing, gossip, and suspects were abounding. Many people *thought* they knew who the guilty party was-creating hard feelings among the congregation. All everyone wanted was for the guilty person to admit their guilt and pay the monies back.

The police were called in to investigate, polygraphs were taken by several people, and one or two people did not pass the polygraph, but, would not admit to any wrong doing. There wasn't an admission nor was there any real any evidence to confirm who actually borrowed the monies; therefore, no one could be charged in the theft. However, the financial books were found to be a mess. The church hired a private investigation team to help get the finances back in line with some checks and balances and hopefully find the missing money and the guilty party. Sounds like a "Who done it?" mystery doesn't it?

During the investigation and turmoil my friends and church were being split right down the middle. People were angry, they were hurt, their trust and faith were wavering. This time period was very upsetting and stressful for most of the congregation. We all wanted an answer to our mystery and a guilty party! Our money back!

Who took the money? The question we all had was; do we continue to give money to the church when the culprit is still in our midst. How was our money being handled and who was handling it? We were taught the monies belonged to God. Who would take from God? Who wouldn't fess up? I understand someone working with the script program probably did *borrow* small amounts of money each time with every intention of returning it. However, the overall amount got out of hand making it impossible to pay back. That was my theory.

Anyway, that Sunday morning in December, 2005 or January, 2006 while we were standing in the balcony overlooking the congregation and I said a prayer. A prayer not like one I had ever said before. I asked God to provide Trinity Church with a hands-on, physical *miracle*. I felt there was a need for a miracle we could see and touch. Miracles happen every day but society is oblivious to them. They are considered coincidences, luck, or just happenstance. I asked God to provide the type of *miracle* that would bring the congregation back to absolute faith in Him. A miracle that would show us God was still in our church working, guiding, and loving us-leaving no room for doubt. I knew in my mind what I wanted God to do. The miracle had to be something no one could question and I prayed to God for that very miracle.

My prayer was for a very active and well known lady in our congregation. She had been fighting esophageal cancer for maybe three years and was about to go into surgery again. Our Pastor was praying for a successful surgical outcome, God's mercy and His will be done. In my great wisdom, I thought if God would just heal this woman and her surgery came out a complete success that would be a perfect hands-on *miracle*. And, it would be a *miracle!*

Most of our active congregation knew this lady and, her husband. They were loved by everyone. A healing miracle of that magnitude would certainly bring people back to unwavering faith, wouldn't it? I thought so. I left the church that morning feeling pretty good; however, I do recall telling God I knew the answer to my prayer was totally up to Him. Whatever His decision, it would be okay with me. Of course His decision would be okay with me! After all, He is God!

In February, 2006 the lady with esophageal cancer died. Needless to say, I was disappointed that God decided to take her home to be with Him rather than use her healing as the miracle I had asked Him for. Honestly though, her passing was a blessing for her and her family. She had been sick for a long time and had endured quite a bit. I'm sure she was tired-I knew she was ready to go live with the Lord. I thanked God for listening and that I understood. I knew He had a different, much better plan, but, I thought I'd ask anyway. Couldn't hurt, right?

Months went by and the controversy continued at church. It was getting hard to attend our regular service with an open mind-too much talk and accusations. It was terrible! Yakity yak all the time! Wayne and I decided to try a different service. We were in hopes there would be more praise and less talk with a different set of worshippers. People we didn't regularly worship with. Trinity was experimenting with a contemporary service on Sunday evenings at 6:00 p.m., and we really do like the contemporary music. So, that's where we were going when the accident occurred. God's miracles began working that day and have continued to work in our lives. He has led me and Wayne on an extraordinarily fulfilling path. Thank you, Lord.

Chapter IV

I could hear Wayne's voice, "Don't move, don't move, you've been in a motorcycle accident. You're in the hospital and you have a trach so don't try to talk. The Pastor is here, can you see him?" I opened my eyes and saw our Pastor smiling at me with his big smile, and white teeth. I nodded and went back to sleep. I tried to wake up; but, it was hard coming out of the coma. I'm not sure I remember everything correctly. I couldn't stay awake for long periods of time, especially at first. I thought I was sleeping; but, my mind seemed to be running all the time. I would wake up just long enough to get bits and pieces of what was going on around me. Wayne wouldn't tell me anything. He was definitely being very protective. More protective than I had ever known him to be. Every time I opened my eyes he was there either standing or sitting in the room watching me–alone. It seemed I was becoming more alert. I looked around the room: it was a typical hospital room; lots of windows on my right, machines on my right, curtain on my left, TV and door at the foot of the bed. I thought I was in the room by myself, but I didn't know for sure. I dozed in and out of sleep. I could see it was dark outside and Wayne had gone home for the evening. I heard people talking on the other side of the curtain next to my bed. It almost sounded as if there was some kind of staff meeting going on. I thought I recognized one voice-a male-the therapy supervisor. Maybe they weren't talking about me; maybe I was sharing the room with someone else. Maybe the voices were visitors for that person. I had a hard time comprehending what I heard. Everything was so confusing! The nice young man returned to my room and that was when I realized he was actually a nurse! He came around my bed and asked if I would like a bath. I smiled and shook my head *yes*. I still couldn't talk. I did want a bath; hadn't had one in I couldn't remember how long. I was ready to get out of that bed and get a shower! What in the world was I thinking? Smiley had a pan of water, soap, wash cloth, and towels sitting on my bedside table. I wasn't getting out of bed after all! For the first time since the accident, I got a look at my body--what I could see of it. I remember thinking, *there's not much to wash.* I had bandages from one end to the other. My lower legs were both wrapped from knees to toes, my arms were both wrapped. The right elbow to fingertips and the left from shoulder to fingertips. There was an incision down my middle running from just under my rib cage all the way down my stomach to just above the hair line. I tried to see what was on the outside of my left leg; because it looked very red, very long, very wide and very open. My leg looked as though there was a piece of raw meat lying against it. In reality, it was a deep, one inch wide thirteen inch long gash; where the bones had popped through the skin. *Oh My! I'm a mess!* I didn't have any pain though. *Couldn't have been that bad without some kind of pain, right?* I felt as if I was in a daze. The bath was over my hospital gown was back on and I didn't remember having been washed. I was preoccupied looking at all my injuries. I was bundled up like a mummy and still pretty much out of it. My head was swimming, from medication. I had tubes everywhere-running up my nose and into my stomach for nourishment, an IV stuck in my arm a PIC line in my neck, a catheter, plus the trach. I couldn't have anything by mouth and my mouth was so dry! I could suck on wet sponges to give moisture to my lips and tongue; but, that was it. Certainly, that wasn't good enough. I was thirsty! *Give me water!* I couldn't have liquids. I might aspirate.

At that point, I didn't know what day it was, how long I had been in the hospital or in the coma. There was a nurse standing behind and to the side of Wayne and he tried to tell me who she was. I remember her being real short, stocky, with short dark brown wavy hair. I nodded my head to acknowledge that I understood what he was saying. She would be taking care of me while I'm in the hospital. I thought, *Okay, I'm good with that. What else was I going to do?*

The hospital can be pretty boring when you are wrapped up like a mummy and on mega pain medication. Wayne was trying to converse with me and that was wonderful. He showed me the flowers and cards I had received from friends. While I was in the coma people had been visiting; but, I was unaware of their presence. A lady friend from church brought in a music tape for me to listen to. However, I don't remember the music.

Ironically, even though I was in a coma, I could hear what was going on around me. That was why our lady friend brought in the music. It was a tool the hospital personnel told my husband to bring in. I could listen to the music and, hopefully, it would encourage me to keep the will to survive. It is strange that I don't remember the music.

Wayne told me a couple of my co-workers wanted to visit and they were waiting until I woke up and was more cognizant to carry on a conversation. I believe they were afraid of what my appearance might be. It was wonderful that everyone had me in their prayers. They chose not to visit right away, which probably was a good thing. Seeing me to soon after the accident would have been quite a shock. My granddaughter, Brandi, said the first time she came to the hospital was very upsetting for her because of all the bruising and swelling. I didn't look like her grandma. She couldn't stay in the room without crying and she had to leave.

I was spacey for the first few weeks after coming out of the coma; people came to visit anyway. I understood the conversations, to a point. I couldn't talk, but I could stay awake. I couldn't tell how much time had passed. I felt like I just existed. I don't remember thinking about eating, going to the bathroom, brushing my teeth, combing my hair, getting dressed, or anything.

One day I opened my eyes to my nurse and someone else rolling me around in the bed. I didn't understand what was happening and I sat up. At least, I thought I sat up. In my head I had asked what they were doing. I couldn't figure it out. Maybe they had given me a bath or changed my bed—anyway, my nurse came stomping around the end of the bed and she yelled at me, "I don't know…Who do you think you are?!" She muttered other words; but, I didn't know what she was talking about, or what I did to upset her. Oh Boy, her comment irritated me. If I had been able to talk, she would have gotten a piece of my mind! I gave her that look--you know the kind. At that moment, I could see she understood I did not like her much. This was just the beginning of my not caring for her. I wanted another nurse assigned to me already. I did not like being talked to the way she had--it was totally uncalled for. Plus, I was unable to tell anyone how she acted or what she said. All I could do was give dirty looks, and, no one knew what they meant.

At shift change, a different nurse came in to introduce herself to us. This lady was tall, average build, long blonde hair pulled back off her face-very friendly. When I looked at her, I thought she was the wife of a probation officer I worked with. I thought he told me she worked in the medical field. *Could it be?!* It would be great if she were who I thought she was. I met her once. She was a young mother of six children-very pleasant and a Christian. I couldn't talk and I couldn't ask her if she was who I thought she was. I had hoped she would stay around. No such luck! She talked to us for a while and left. I saw her a few more times--on different days. Anyway, it turned out she wasn't who I first thought she was. My feelings of well being disappeared.

My morphine dreams/thoughts were unusual, complicated, and scary, to say the least. My mind drifted into those dreams quite often during my time in the coma. One of those times happened when, in my mind, I was taken to an unknown location for unknown reasons with the nurse I did not trust.

Help! She's back and she's taking me someplace without my husband! I thought I was loaded into a vehicle and driven to a place by the ocean-a beautiful chalet on the beach. Someone got me out of the vehicle and took me inside a building. I'm confused, *what's going on?* Seems like an open house of some sort. *What am I doing here?!* I was laid on a bed in a room by myself, with a curtain to my left. I can hear a lot of people talking and laughing. I think it's about me, but, I can't make it out. People I don't know come over to my side of the room, look at me then leave as if I'm on display. *Tell me something! What is going on?* My nurse came in to check on me. I will not respond to her. I'm upset with her and a little afraid. Because of my trach, I can't tell anyone what she said to me or ask why she said, *"Who do you think you are?"* I couldn't defend myself either, if I had to. I guess I'm worried about what else she might do or say.

She told me to stay where I was and not move. *Don't know where I'd go, I don't know where I am!* An older man and woman introduce themselves to me as proprietors of the building. I don't know anything about them or why they're even talking to me. They have given me the impression the get together was for their retirement.

I hear a voice I recognize! It's the probation officer from work; the guy whose wife I thought was my other nurse. I had a hard time getting up to look around the curtain. *It's him!* I needed to get his attention and hopefully he would get me out of that place or get a message to Wayne. I didn't think he knew where I was. He came in, said *hello* and asked how I felt. My nurse was with him. She's all smiles and friendly. I looked at her thinking, *what is going on?!* I can't say anything to him. My chance was lost. What's the matter with me, *I can't talk. I have a trach!* My nurse left. She said she was helping with the food and she'll return later. *I wouldn't let her near the food! I wish I could get it across to someone that I don't like it here. I want to go home! People are leaving-I'm alone with my nurse again. Okay, I hear Wayne he found me! I'm leaving too! I hope. Yeah! Don't leave me, Wayne, take me with you! I don't want to be alone with that nurse! I don't trust her.*

I felt as if someone was pushing me in a wheel chair. *It's Wayne!* He's taking me away from the chalet by the ocean. I was so glad; I didn't know why I was there in the first place. I could see the beach area as we left: The waves crashing over the rocks; and, the scrub brush here and there. The sun was shining, the sky was blue, there were some white, fluffy clouds floating by. It looked beautiful; and it was all just in my mind.

I thought I had been transported to a nursing home or hospital, I couldn't tell for sure. I was in a hallway with lots of people hustling and bustling all around me. The surroundings seemed very pleasant. Wayne was talking to different nurses. Some of the nurses were talking very caringly to me. I could not comprehend exactly what was being said. One nurse told me I'd be okay that they would take good care of me-not to worry. Wayne told them my nurse and I was not getting along very well. Everyone said they understood.

My nurse didn't seem to have the reputation of an easy nurse to get along with. *Surprise, Surprise!* The comments I heard were not good about her and I understood them to say they were going to replace her as my nurse. *I'm all for that!*

The conversation continued and whatever was said; I got the feeling, I was headed for surgery, tests, or something. Wayne walked along side me as I was pushed down a hallway by a nurse. I thought we were going to my room; then, I drifted off again.

I woke up and realized I had been wheeled to someplace else. *Now where are they taking me?* I was going down a long plain looking hallway, around a corner and into a gray room full of equipment. I didn't see Wayne--he wasn't there. I felt very uncomfortable. No one told me anything! It was as if they thought I didn't have the *need to know* what was going. I was in a coma anyway. Little did they understand that I could see and hear them talking. They were moving the equipment around in the room; it seemed like a storage room with surgery equipment stored there. I didn't like that. Everyone I saw in the room had a very sober look on their face. No one was talking and when they did talk, I couldn't hear what was being said. It was very quiet. I had been moved onto some kind of cold table. I was turned onto my left side; positioned, and repositioned. I needed to be just right for whatever was going to happen. A nurse put a warm blanket on me-it was cold in that room, whatever that room was. I saw a man with a white jacket on and gloves-he could have been a doctor. He was average height, short reddish-blonde hair, and light complexion with freckles. *Is he a doctor?* He was pretty brash and unprofessional to the other people in the room- almost to the point of being rude. *Oh great! This man is going to do something to me!* He had some kind of a long wire, like an opened up coat hanger, in his hands. He pushed and pulled on me attempting to put the wire in my right ear. He pushed and pulled some more; but, the wire wouldn't go in my ear. He kept pushing--*that hurt! Stop! Please, stop!* Out of the corner of my eye I could see a lady and a man standing off to the side. They both looked solemn as they watched. The doctor working on me had absolutely no compassion. He treated me as if I was a lifeless body lying there. *Why didn't the other two stop him?* I wanted to reach out to them; but, I couldn't move. I heard him ask them what they thought and they said they didn't know. *I'm in pain!* Finally, there were tears coming from my eyes. *Maybe they'll see my tears and make him stop.* Whoever this guy was, he asked the other two people again what they thought. They conversed some about him stopping and leaving things alone. Finally, he did stop. They moved me from the table back onto the gurney and a transporter took me out the doors and down the hall. *Good!* I'm relieved.

I can't breathe! I can't breathe! I can't catch my breath! My breathing passage was plugged. I pounded on my chest struggling to breathe! *Help! I can't sit up! I can't breathe!* I tried tipping my head back to see who was pushing me to get his attention. *Look! I can't breathe!* There was an older black man, balding, average stature, dressed in scrubs pushing the gurney. He looked at me asking, "What's wrong? Are you alright?" *NO! I can't breathe! I'm pounding on my chest! Can't you see what I'm doing?!* He stopped the cart, casually walked up along side of me, looked at me, and said, "Oh My! You can't breathe?! Hold on! I'll get you help!" He ran back to the end of the cart and started pushing; quickly this time. I laid there, looked up at the ceiling, relaxed, and stopped pounding on my chest. I prayed, *God, I'm in your hands. I can't do anymore.* Instantaneously, thoughts of my husband, daughter, and granddaughters ran through my head. I thought I won't ever see them again. Then, I thought, they would be alright. God would take care of them and I continued with my prayer, *if this is my time to come live with you, I guess, I'm ready.* A few seconds later the plug popped! *I can breathe! Thank you, God! I can breathe!* The transporter pushed me quickly around another corner, and then there was another lapse of time. I was in and out of consciousness; but, I could hear the nurses all around me, talking and complaining. They were angry. They were talking about a doctor they didn't think should have been doing whatever procedure he had done on me. "He's not suited!" They did not like his demeanor. One of the nurses said they almost lost me to the motorcycle accident and then to a stroke. I couldn't understand what else she said. The ladies fussed around me like a baby; wrapped me up, turned me from side to side, and covered me. They were very gentle and they were very irritated at the same time. I just took it all in; even though, I really was not sure what they were talking about or even doing. The medication created mass confusion in my head.

Chapter V

Aprell visited; but, she didn't bring my granddaughters every time. They were young; Brandi, age 14; and Brittany, age 8. She brought Brandi once and that was enough. The accident had been a very traumatic incident for both girls. When Brandi saw me the first time she knew it would be extremely hard for the two of them to handle. Brittany was too young and Aprell didn't allow her to visit. She didn't want Brittany to see me in the state I was in.

Aprell and I had a good visit; however, when it was time for her to leave, I started getting anxious and I didn't want her to leave. I couldn't tell her why I was scared. Every time my visitors left I would go for more tests. I begged, in my silent way, for my daughter not to leave. It was getting late and she couldn't stay. I observed the look of worry and fear in her eyes. She knew I wanted to say something and couldn't. I had to stop fussing and let her go home to her girls. Aprell left and just as I thought, the transporters came in to transport me for more tests.

I didn't know why I was moved. I laid in the fetal position on a bed in another room, which appeared to be a kind of doctor's office. There was a receptionist who directed patients to different rooms just like in a doctor's office. I lay on the bed and watched. I did not move. It hurt to move. I was talking to another lady in the same room.. She was there for tests too. We seemed to lay for a long time with no doctor. We were told he would be there after he completed tasks elsewhere. I didn't know how much time passed-seemed like an eternity. I was so achy, my body hurt all over. The atmosphere surrounding me and the other lady seemed not quite right. A nurse put a warm cover over me. I was chilled and I felt like I had the flu or something. There was a lot of conversation all around me. I didn't know what it was about. It sounded illegal, like drug transactions or something. The doctor came into the room with his expensive suit on and he flitted around the room. He looked at me and the other lady then walked away from us. He acted as if he thought he was 'God's gift to the world'; but, something was not right. I felt too sick to care. I could hear talk about morphine and other drugs. I also heard a pretty heated discussion between the doctor and another man. The nurse who covered me said he should be arrested. He had no business doing what he did-she was not talking to me.. She told me to lay quiet and it would be okay. This was so weird; I thought I was in an opiate den. It was so dark and smoky gray, with an eerie atmosphere. There were beads hanging between me, the receptionist and the other patient. The air was smoke filled and hazy. *What am I doing here?! Who was this doctor they brought me to?!* All of a sudden the door opened forcefully. A group of men charged in, grabbed the doctor, pushed him over a chair from the waist up, handcuffed him and took him away. The nurse, who had been taking care of me, commented that it was all over. She had done the right thing and we would be alright. I was still in the fetal position and I still hurt. I was at peace though. I was taken from that room and returned to my bed in my room. What an experience that was-at least in my head. My pain meds are playing with my mind. My dreams were quite dreadful.

I was oblivious to the passing of time. After a while, my head seemed to clear some. I could sit up in bed, with the help of the bed and pillows. The bed would roll me from one side to the other I could feel rollers underneath me moving from the head of the bed to the foot-this kept me moving and stopped me from developing bed sores. I couldn't move myself so the bed did it for me. I had a trach in my throat and couldn't talk. My hands were wrapped and I couldn't write. Communication was very difficult. Wayne was not good at reading my lips or deciphering my expressions. He did pick up on my angry looks; but, he couldn't figure out what I was angry about. I couldn't tell him what went on after he would leave. It didn't matter at that point anyway.

My mother-in-law visited often. My brother-in-law would bring her because of the distance she would have to drive by herself. She brought me a Prayer Shawl, made by a lady at a Lutheran Church in Ida, Mi. The lady wasn't from our church; but, news travels fast in a small community and the lady knew my mother-in-law. The shawl was very pretty and the prayers were very much appreciated. My mother-in-law took the shawl home with her until I could come home. We didn't want to leave anything in my room because it could come up missing or get messed up. I certainly couldn't keep track of anything. My husband lost it once with the nurses on the floor because of the lack of tidiness in my room. The nurses would come in, do their thing, throw stuff on the floor or around the room and leave it for the housekeeping staff to clean up. "Not my job, man!" You know how that goes.

No one has told me what exactly happened. I know I was in a motorcycle accident and it must have been bad; but, I hadn't comprehended just how bad. I was told it was very important for me to get all the rest I could. A nurse or CNA entered my room and told me how she tried to comb my hair. It was snarled and had blood in it. She said she got most of the blood out; but, she had to cut a clump of hair off in the back because it was too matted to comb out. She said she used to be a beautician and she was careful. She told me not to worry no one would see it and hair always grows back. I smiled and nodded. In my head, I told her I was alright with her combing and cutting my hair. I was silently delighted that someone was attending to my hair.

During the night I opened my eyes to a young lady; short in stature, thin with long, wavy, dark brown hair hanging over her shoulders. She was leaning over me-almost in my face. Her right hand was up by my neck. I startle her and she jumped back from me pulling her arm/hand back freaking out, "I didn't do anything, I didn't do anything, really, I didn't!" I couldn't tell her that it was okay. I tried to reach out to her to let her know I wasn't accusing her of anything. She stood there, not moving, just watching me. I drifted off, shutting my eyes for a second. When I opened them again; she was leaning over me again with her hand back up by my neck. She saw my eyes open and she jumped back a second time, saying, "I'm not doing anything, really, I'm not". I nodded my head to let her know she was okay. She moved back farther away from me this time. I thought it was a little odd, her being there so close to me; but, I was tired. I shut my eyes briefly for a third time. I opened them again and she was gone. I couldn't help but wonder what she was doing or what she was going to do. And, why did I wake up at the exact time she reached out to me--twice. She hadn't touched me to disturb me. I didn't have any jewelry on. The only thing on my neck was the trach and a pick line. She appeared to be an employee of the hospital. She had a name tag hanging around her neck. I couldn't see her name and she was wearing dark blue scrubs. It seemed strange that her long hair was down and not put up. I hadn't seen her before and I never saw her again. Who she was and what was she doing. I'll never know. However, I do know angels were around me, both good and bad.

Chapter VI

Days come and go; I thought I was getting better. There seemed to be a lot of things going on in my head and some of them didn't make a lot of sense to me. I was sitting in bed with Wayne in the room visiting me when three men walked in. They were standing at the foot of my bed just looking at me–*this is weird.* I looked at Wayne, he looked at me and we both looked back at the three men. It was funny. Finally, Wayne said, "this is the doctor who put you back together". I turned and looked at the three men. I had no clue who was who. I smiled. They didn't say anything; just stood there then turned and left! *Well, Okay!* Wayne pointed out that the orthopedic doctor was the man in the middle and his two interns were on either side of him. They were the orthopedic team that worked on me. When I think of them now-standing there, I think of Shadrach, Meshach and Abednego before being thrown into the fiery furnace. Only, the operating room with me was their fiery furnace. What a nightmare--for them!

The next day, after the doctor and his interns visited, I was taken down to the doctor-patient examining rooms for an examination of my wounds. An intern started changing the wound vacs on my legs. Now, if you don't know about wound vacs; they work similar to vacuum cleaners. Sponges are cut to fit exactly inside an open wound, tubing is put on top of the sponges and taped in place-air tight. The tape is placed over the sponges as well and-in my case-around my legs. When the vacuum machine is turned on, the air is sucked up out of the sponges along with any dead tissue from inside the wounds; that promotes quicker healing. Back to the intern, he didn't tell me what he was about to do he just started pulling the tape off my leg. It felt as if he was pulling duck tape off my legs! I couldn't say anything, but I must have been doing a bit of squirming and grimacing. The intern looked at me and said, "Oh, stop that! It doesn't hurt that bad, you don't need to act like that." I shot him a look! I was thinking, *Let me pull tape off your hairy legs and see how you react! I'm sorry, but, it did hurt!* To this day hair does not grow on my legs.

Right after that intern changed my wound vacs, I was laying quietly on the gurney when another intern walked up. He looked at the skin graph on my right leg and without warning, he pulled off the scabs. I shot him a *look* too. He would not look at me. A third intern told me, "its okay that black has to come off." Whatever black he was talking about. A little heads up sure would have been nice.

A fourth intern was sitting to my left picking at the scabs around the stitches on my upper left arm when he said, "This hole in your elbow will never heal, you will always have a hole here. That can't be fixed." I thought to myself, *what is this, torture Sandy day?* I still remember the faces of these four interns, not their names, but their faces. I thought, these boys needed to be on the other side of the gurney once. I couldn't say what I was really thinking; but, I definitely felt what they did and heard what they said.

The next day, another group of young interns entered my room. These young interns were there to take out my trach tubing. I didn't know how long the trach had been there, but, I was very happy to be getting rid of it. One intern reassured me taking the trach out would not hurt. He was right-no pain. He asked me to say something while he put his finger over the hole in my neck. I believe my first word was "Hi". The nurses and aides that were watching actually clapped and cheered. I didn't quite understand all the excitement; but, I was smiling from ear to ear. The intern told me the hole would heal quickly. In the meantime, I needed to close it off with my finger to talk. *No problem,! Thank you! Praise God! Look out my favorite nurse-not!*

The doctor's physician assistant was the only person left in the room with me. I had seen her once before; but, I couldn't remember her name. She was ecstatic over hearing my voice. She was so excited she said, "You need to call your husband and talk to him. Where's your phone? No phone, I will find you one, I'll be right back." She left and returned with a phone. She ran around my room looking for a plug in and couldn't find one. I tried to tell her Wayne would hear me talk when he came to visit. She stopped, finally, leaned over the railing of my bed and told me why she wanted me to call Wayne. She said, "I wanted you to call him, because a while ago I made a call to your home. The answering machine came on-she began to cry-your voice was on the answering machine…she paused…your voice sounded so soft and sweet. You are a miracle." I reassured her it was okay, Wayne would hear me talk before the day ended. I did not understand why it was so important to them that I got my voice back. I didn't feel I was any different than any other patient in the hospital. I was still me, banged up and bruised; but, me. I guess, I didn't see the whole picture. As for being a *miracle*, I didn't know about that either.

I looked up and there was another friendly face. I smiled and said, "Hello". The young male nurse his tracks, gasped, put his hand up by his mouth, and said, "You're talking!" Oh, my gosh! Say it again!" I said, "Hello", again. He came over to me and said, "I can't believe it! Your voice! It's not what I thought you would sound like! I'm so excited! I thought you would sound…I don't know…not what you sound like. You know how you get an idea in your head of what people look like from the way they sound. I got an idea of what you would sound like from the way you look. My idea didn't match. Your voice is so much softer." I wondered what he thought I would sound like; maybe a deep raspy biker babe voice. Funny! Smiley was on duty so he couldn't stay and talk; however, when Wayne arrived, he came back to my room for a while before he went home. It had been an exciting day and I was worn out.

I was lying on my left side and I thought I had been asleep. I opened my eyes and saw a young man at my bedside. He was short, about 5 feet 5 inches tall, light brown curly hair, wearing dark blue scrubs, name tag, and he had a stethoscope around his neck. He was acting nervous. I looked at him and he looked at me. He said nothing at first, then, "I'm here for your trach". I smiled and nodded. I knew I could speak, but, I'm tired. Then he said, "I'm your guardian angel". I looked at him a little harder, and I thought, *I should ask him his name-Are you Gabriel?* But, I was too tired. I just thought; *okay, he said he was my angel* and that was good enough. I looked up again and he was gone. I never saw him before and I never saw him again. I thought later my trach was out. Why was he on my left side, when all the machines were on my right side. The curtain on my left side was pulled back when he was there and I didn't hear him open or close it. If I'm dreaming, this all seemed very real to me.

Chapter VII

All my days ran together. Wayne said he told some of our friends that I could have visitors. I hoped I could stay awake long enough to talk to them. I felt pretty punchy. Some days I felt punchier than others; but, I thought I was up to talking.

A couple of probation officers I worked with stopped by and brought me flowers and a card. I appreciated seeing them, it was great! They didn't stay long. They told me my accident was bad-very bad-and the rumors were flying. One rumor was that I had lost my left leg. Not true, yet, anyway. They said they would go back to work and give an actual account of my condition. I sensed they were concerned. They said the accident was the worst the police officers had seen in a while. In fact, for a new officer on the scene, it was down right eye opening. He wasn't exactly prepared for the extensive injuries I had. He had to take some time off work to process the accident and the severity of the injuries. My co-workers were pulling for me and praying for my recovery. As the ladies were leaving, they said for me to take care and that they would be back to see me soon. I was so glad to talk to them-really glad.

My next set of visitors was my stepdaughter and her husband. This was a surprise! They were standing on my left side; no one ever sat down and stayed for any length of time. Wayne's daughter said, "I knew something bad was wrong when Dad called, he was crying and I've never heard him cry before". I looked at her and I wanted to say something; but, I didn't. I was polite. I smiled and said, "He was?" There's been a bit of muddy water under that bridge and most of it had been muddied up by divorce; but, that was another story.

A motorcycle friend of ours from church visited several times, while I was in the coma. He was a Christian guy married to a real nice Christian gal. I liked them both. He told Wayne was going to get him a *bell* for his bike. (A bell attached to a motorcycle signifies good luck.) That was a real nice gesture. . He also told us his wife sold her bike. My accident scared her. I was very sorry to hear she didn't want to ride anymore. If she liked riding, she should ride. We found out later that another rider friend from church sold his bike for the same reason--my accident.

I love Aprell. She came back to see me. We could actually talk; I have my voice back. I asked her about the accident-what had happened. I wanted to know. She told me some and left out a lot. I did get a better idea of what had happened though. She briefly told me: as I was going into a curve, I ran head-on into an oncoming vehicle. The bike was totaled. No one was ticketed. I was the only victim. My injuries were life threatening. I was flown by the Life-Flite helicopter to the trauma unit at a hospital in Toledo, Ohio. The hospital staff was on alert and prepared for my arrival. They cleaned my wounds the best they could; took some x-rays, did a CT scan, gave me eight pints of blood, operated, took out my spleen, bandaged all my wounds, and put me in a medically induced coma for at least three weeks. I digested that information to a point. It was a lot of information and not good, but, I had to begin to deal with it. Aprell said she and the girls would be around and Dad would keep them up to date, if she couldn't make it down to see me. I began to think I wasn't going home soon. There must have been more to my story; but, at the moment I didn't think I would be able to absorb more. The information was not totally registering as it should've, and maybe I was blocking it out. I don't know. Things just were not feeling right. I felt numb.

Chapter VIII

The beginning of an extremely long healing process had already begun. The first three or four weeks were more of a waiting period; they were waiting for me to stabilize. I did not realize how much I was actually going through.

Four weeks after the accident, the major operation was in the making. I was aware of an operation; just not aware of how serious it was going to be. Wayne and I were waiting in pre-op, and I acted as if I didn't have a concern in the world. The date was June 22, 2006. I was prepped for the operation by the nurses and the anesthesiologist. They asked questions upon questions. The IV was filling my bladder with water and it seemed I needed a bed pan every few minutes. Wayne was sitting in a chair on my left, leaning on the railing. It must have been early in the morning, because he was having a hard time staying awake or maybe it was probably the stress. A nurse came over and asked me what they were operating on. I told her my legs; and, she marked both legs with a marker. Wayne questioned what she was doing and she stated it was a precaution. Insuring everything went right in the operating room and they operated on the right parts. I didn't realize it was going to be *both* legs. Next, I talked to the interns who were assisting the ortho doctor. The worst part was the time spent waiting; it seemed like hours and hours. A young man came with a needle and some medicine that would make me drowsy and relaxed before I went into surgery. That was nice; I liked being relaxed. It must be time to go, the surgery nurse came in. She introduced herself to us and made sure I had on my surgery booties and hat. She told me and Wayne to kiss, hug so-long and see *ya* later. She pulled me out of the waiting area and Wayne told them to bring me back, "bring her back--alive". I thought he was kidding. The nurse said, "Oh yeah, she'll be okay, we will take good care of her and we'll bring her back soon" then she turned and looked at Wayne. I couldn't see Wayne, but, whatever he was doing wasn't good. The look on the nurse's face went from happy to very dark and serious. I wanted to get up, turn around and see what was going on, but, I didn't--probably a good thing. They wheeled me through the first set of doors and then the second set. It got cold--like an icebox. By the time we arrived at the operating room door, I could hardly keep my eyes open. There were several people flitting around doing one thing or another. Some of them stopped what they were doing, grabbed the sheet I was laying on and pulled me over to the table; then the nurse strapped my arms down. That was not a good feeling--helpless. I felt panicky. The anesthesiologist told me that after I went to sleep, he would put a tube down my throat to keep me breathing and asleep. I was glad he took the time to explain to me what was happening. He put a plastic mask over my nose and mouth; then he told me to count back from ten. I got to eight--lights out. That was easy.

Somebody slapped me on the face and called my name. "Sandy, Sandy, it's time to wake up. Come on now. Wake up. How do you feel?" I was in *PAIN!!!* Lots of *PAIN!* Excruciating *PAIN!* I screamed, "Make it stop! It hurts!" I had never felt pain like that before! My nurse stood on my right side, very serious and calm. I asked her to give me something to stop the pain, "Please! It hurts!" She said she had just given me something. I couldn't wait. I called out to God, "God, please stop the pain! Jesus, please, it hurts!" The nurse said, "I'm giving you morphine and I need to wait at least five minutes before I can give you any more." I sighed and drifted off; but, not for very long. The pain woke me up. I asked for Wayne and was told he couldn't come to me yet. The nurse told me I didn't want him to see me in so much pain. After a few minutes,

Wayne came in. He looked so tired; but, he tried to be upbeat. He smiled at me, took my hand, and asked how I was doing. I was hurting; but, I wasn't getting sick to my stomach--that was a good thing. The morphine finally kicked in and the pain was not as great as it was. My legs were bandaged and there was an external fixator on my left leg holding the bones in place. I had never seen a fixator like that before. All the metal it looked like an erector set on the outside of my leg. Apparently, external fixators hold bones in place better than casts. I was a little hungry; but, I could only have crackers and 7-Up. I didn't remember going back to my room nor did I remember the rest of the day or that night. About three years later, I was going through some paperwork and found a list of procedures that was done during the operation on June 22, 2006. The words *cardiac arrest* jumped out at me. That was interesting; no one told me or Wayne that my heart stopped during that surgery; but, they brought me back *alive* under the supervision of the Greatest Physician of all--God.

Later on, in my room, I recognized a CNA fussing around, picking up things and straightening up. I recognized her by her long, brown, thick, braided ponytail lying down on her back. I thought her hair was really pretty. She either thought I was sleeping or she didn't realize I could talk, because she was quietly going about doing her job when I said "hello". I startled her, and then we started talking. She asked me, "Do you remember me last night standing at the foot of your bed while you were sleeping? I stood there holding your foot--crying. I felt so helpless and sorry for you." She didn't know why her emotions came over her like that. She said she cried and prayed for me. I thanked her from the bottom of my heart. What a wonderful gesture, for no reason and for someone she didn't know. I saw her once or twice after that, but, we never really talked again. I won't forget what she did though. Praise God.

A few nights later, I talked with another CNA that was in my room picking up and she said she thought she remembered me when I came into the hospital. She wasn't sure it was me though. The lady she saw was swollen and black and blue, but, the lady had been a motorcycle accident victim. After a little more conversation, we concluded I was the lady she saw come in and the change in my appearance was remarkable.

Within a few days of my last operation, Wayne and the hospital staff were trying to locate a nursing home for me to be transferred to so I could continue recuperating. It had to be a place that could handle everything I had going on and believe me there was a whole lot going on with me. Besides all the tubes going everywhere, there were wound vacs on both my legs which needed to be changed every three or four days, open wounds that needed bandage changes daily, a skin graph on my right leg that needed to be watched for infection, etc, etc, etc. Anyway, most nursing homes were not set up for that extensive of care, because they don't do it very often. I was going to be a refresher course for most nursing home nurses. Not to mention it was a learning experience for me and my husband. After a bit of discussion, it was decided I would go to Parkside Nursing Home in Toledo, Ohio. The next day I was transported via ambulance to Parkside.

My arrival was anticipated by the nursing staff; and, Wayne was waiting as well. Everyone seemed friendly enough. The building was old, the hallways were narrow, and I was on the fifth floor. The room was actually very nice, small, but nice with a private bathroom-that I couldn't use. It seemed pretty homey, I could not see out into the hallway because of the position of the bed. The staff seemed to be receptive of my coming into their facility even with all my problems. They said I was a refreshing change from their usual patients.

My morning CNA was a good caretaker. She did everything she could helping me be comfortable; even washed my hair with real water! Boy that felt good! Especially after six weeks of not having had my hair washed. Along with all my physical problems, I was having hot flashes and my CNA searched the floors for a fan. I was extremely grateful to her for finding one. She was a good lady.

My afternoon CNA was an older, black lady who getting close to retirement. At first she was friendly and helpful; however, she turned out to be pretty grumpy especially after Wayne would go home in the evening. She complained that I had to pee too often and I needed the bed pan which she had to get for me. Well, I was taking a water pill and I had an IV putting fluids back into me. Those two items might have had something to do with my need to urinate often. Plus, I needed to be turned or moved to prevent bed sores, and she didn't care for that either because she could not do it by herself. She needed to look for someone to help her every time I had to be moved.

The midnight crew was a *different* crew. My midnight CNA was a male who was not very talkative or friendly. He did his job and would not go an extra inch for anything or anyone. I remember asking him if he would arrange for me to get my breakfast earlier than normal as I had an early morning doctor appointment. He informed me that getting my breakfast was up to the morning shift, not him and if they didn't get it to me before I had to leave--I didn't eat. He wouldn't give me an early bath or help me brush my teeth either. Those responsibilities were the morning shifts responsibilities. I would go to the doctor early and return after lunch without being washed or having eaten. More often than not, when I returned my bed wasn't made. The EMTS people would make it so they could put me in it and leave. Certainly wasn't their job; but, I was very thankful they took the time. I rode in the ambulance so often I got to know the guys and girls pretty well. They were good to me.

The morning nurse at Parkside was okay, I didn't really see her very often just at med time or when she came in to my room to change my bandages. One morning when she was changing my elbow bandage a young CNA was helping her by supporting my elbow. We were talking and I looked up at the CNA whose eyes were rolling back into her head. She began to fall over on top of me. With my right hand, I grabbed her braids and told the nurse I thought she passed out. My bed was sitting at an angle to the wall and the nurse pushed the CNA, with her hips, up into the wedge between the wall and my bed so she wouldn't fall on the floor. At that point, the CNA woke up, finished helping the nurse, and immediately left for the bathroom. The nurse said that she might want to rethink her career choice--she wanted to be a nurse.

The afternoon nurse was a male, about 5' 8", stocky, red hair, butch hair cut, an ex Navy man, married with six children. Wayne did not care for him for some reason-I didn't know why. I had some problems with him; but, I thought, all in all, he was a good nurse-just opinionated. One night I asked for some kind of medication, don't remember what it was anymore; but, apparently the meds came from the next floor up and the nurse up there had to mix it. Well, by the time she arrived to give it to me I had decided I really didn't need it. She left; the male nurse came into my room and bawled me out for asking for medicine and not taking it. He told me if I wasn't going to take it, not to ask for it. The medicine was time consuming to mix and when she brought it to me; I took the nurse away from her post. I let the chewing out roll off my back; however, a CNA that overheard him didn't. She went to bat for me and told him not to treat me like that; it was my prerogative as a patient to decline the medicine. Later she came to me and told me what she had said to the nurse. He watched her very carefully that night. I hoped she didn't have any problems later on; but, isn't it great how God works. His angels were on guard. The male nurse really was pretty tolerant of me. I think I frustrated him with all I had going on. One night the wound vac on my right leg was beeping continuously. No matter what he did it wouldn't stop. Fed up, he came into my room and said he couldn't take it anymore and turned it off completely. I made a comment about all the other beeping from the other rooms and he said they didn't bother him-just mine. Those other call lights were beeping a whole lot more than mine, and they were people who wanted help of some sort. I was amazed at his comment.

The midnight nurse was a good lady. I hadn't been in the nursing home very long, a couple of day's maybe, when I had my first incident. It was after midnight, I was sleeping, dreaming, and hallucinating all at the same time. For some reason, I thought I was at my daughter's apartment. I was all turned around. I remember talking to Aprell, I was trying to get her attention about the furniture arrangement in her living room. I tried to get out of bed. My legs were all tangled in ropes or something--so I thought. I started fighting and kicking to get untangled. Slipping off the side of the bed I caught myself; realizing I needed help, I yelled for the nurse. When she came into my room, she called for help. She tried to lift my legs and put me back in bed, but, she couldn't get a good hold of me with all the gear attached to my legs. I remember telling her to let me stand up or let me slide all the way off the bed onto the floor so I could stand up. Of course she said "No"! I think I scared both the nurse and the CNA because after that, I had a bed alarm; at least, until the CNA got tired of coming into my room turning it off, because I moved. I was pretty good after that though. I kept myself mindful of my surroundings.

For the most part, Wayne fed me lunch and dinner. The CNAs did everything else when they got around to it. I could not do anything myself which was disheartening for me. I spent all of my spare time watching TV or sleeping. I did have a big support group: my family, friends, and most of all my church. All of those people really pulled together for my husband and me. They pulled together like I hadn't seen them pull together for quite some time. It was wonderful! I had different visitors all the time. I was seeing more and more people from church. People I usually saw only once a week and normally just to say hello to--this was absolutely wonderful!

I did have other visitors too, some that I didn't know. They popped in to talk for a minute then would leave. They were people who worked at the nursing home. One such visitor was, I believe, a housekeeper who stopped to talk for a moment. She related a story of an uncle of hers who had a motorcycle accident at the age of 60. This uncle had been put in a medically induced coma following his accident-the same as me. The man was going to lose a leg and the family decided the victim could not handle the loss of his leg so they let him go--he died. We wondered what motivated people to tell stories like that to people in a similar situation like I was. Wayne sat and looked at me- knowing she did mean well.

I was in mega pain and there was a moment when I thought, *if I just stop eating, this would be all over for me and everyone.* Then my thoughts turned to God and how He had put me in the hands of people who were doing their best to keep me alive; and, then there were all those people who were praying for me. I thought *I can't let God down; He has a reason for this to be happening to me.* I talked to Him all the time. I could remember the Lord's Prayer, which I prayed often; but, I couldn't remember the Doxology. I remembered some of it, but, not all of it. I wanted to recite the Doxology to praise the Lord. I knew His Angels were with me--I could feel them patting the bed covers. I thought someone was in my room; but, when I looked up, no one was there.

I couldn't remember the accident.-I tried and tried. I remembered Wayne going into the curve, I remembered hearing the little voices on my left and right; and, I remembered the pick-up truck in my rear view mirror-that was it. The nurse suggested a psych doctor come into talk to me about my memory of the accident. The doctor told me that trying to remember the accident was fruitless and I probably should not try anymore. The bump on my head basically wiped out my memory of the accident; but, I couldn't help trying, hoping something would return eventually.

There was a team of ladies that came into my room every two or three days to change my wound vacs and bandages. I managed to get a bed sore on my left heel from rubbing my heel on the bed trying to push myself up to the head of the bed. I was moving as much as I could in order not to get any other bed sores-especially on my bottom. I could deal with the one on my heel; there wasn't constant pressure on it. The ladies were very nice and patient with me. I did get impatient with one of them one evening, though. The first time she changed the wound vac on my left leg she had a very hard time getting it to seal. About the third hour, I was getting real tired and so was she. She ended up calling in her supervisor to help her figure out how to get the tape sealed around the fixator bars. Finally, the tape sealed and the wound vac began sucking the way it was supposed to. Praise God!

The therapy team came in to do therapy every few days or so. They really didn't do much at first.. My muscles were gone; my legs were so skinny it was pathetic. Remember that song, 'Who'll take the lady with the skinny legs?' That was me! Anyway, for the first time since the accident, three months prior, therapy tried to set me in a wheelchair. I sat maybe two minutes before I had to lay back down. I was very light headed, shaky, and sick to my stomach. It was amazing how much strength I lost and how quickly I lost it. It was also amazing how little the therapists understood that fact. They thought I could get up and sit in the wheelchair for at least an hour. And when I couldn't sit up for the five minutes they wanted me to, they didn't try getting me up a second time for a week or two. The next time I managed to sit five minutes in the wheelchair.

I began setting up on the edge of the bed and dangling my legs over the side for a few minutes at a time. The blood rushing into my legs caused pressure and a lot of pain; but, I kept sitting a little longer each time. The third time therapy came in, got me up, and put me in the wheelchair; I actually stayed in it for thirty minutes. That was when I got my first real look at the nursing home and the residents. Never having been in a nursing home before but to visit, I can tell you the experience was eye opening. My afternoon CNA said she couldn't wait for me to get up and around; she wanted to take me into the bathroom and outside on the home's grounds. I liked her idea, but, it was going to be a long time down the road before that happened.

As I became more aware of what was going on around me, I moved around a bit more in bed-rearranging myself. Wayne would get after me because I would be leaning on or pulling myself up in bed using my right arm. He knew I had broken that wrist and it had a pin in it. I did not. Therefore, he was afraid I would undo what the doctors had fixed. I told him my wrist didn't hurt and I was fine. He shook his head and walked away.

I wanted to eat real food and drink real water. Tube feeding and thickened liquids were getting very old. Eventually, I convinced the nutritionist to send me to the hospital for a second swallow test. After the first test, I graduated to pureed foods; now, I had to show them I could actually swallow food and not aspirate. I was taken to the hospital where they put me in this chair to be x-rayed. The staff could observe my throat when I swallowed food making sure it went down the right pipe *Okay, I can do this, I'm ready.*

Remember earlier when I talked about a doctor that was rude and not compassionate. He did some sort of test on me, when I was in a coma, that hurt. Well, just before I was given some pudding to eat, in walked that red headed doctor. I remembered him soon as I laid eyes on him; the hair on the back of my neck stood up and I got chills! I was immediately upset. *He had better not come close. I just may have a comment or two for him! Thank the Lord- he left.* I could not believe how I quickly my dander got up when that man came into the room. I do not know for sure what he did to me; but, I know I did not like it! I passed my swallow test despite that doctor upsetting me. Now I could eat real food! However, they were still feeding me at night via a tube; at least a quart of liquid food, maybe not quite that much; but, it sure felt like it. During the day I was told to eat! *You have got to be kidding! Stop the tube feeding and I might have an appetite!* It took a bit of talking, but, I finally got that point across to them and the feeding tube was removed.

Things were still not going right. I was hungry and I wanted to eat, but, the food did not taste good. In fact, it tasted terrible! I had lost quite a bit of weight, which was not good. Wayne tried a carrot salad I had for dinner one afternoon. He said it tasted like paper--I laughed and told him I had been trying to tell him that all along. Salad, fruit, potatoes, and pasta salads were all I ate for a while. Oh, by the way, I was normally a lefty and when I did finally pick up a fork to eat, I used my right hand and thought, *this is weird*. It was awkward and then I realized I was using my right hand instead of my left. I made it work.

I made many trips from Parkside to the hospital for exams, x-rays, and operations; just about every two, four, and six weeks. The hospital personnel knew me and Wayne by our first names without asking. Each of my visits was like visiting old family and friends. I was told a few years later that when I would arrive at the hospital for checkups and x-rays, the technicians would talk amongst each other; "Sandra's here…how's she doing…what does she look like…is she okay?" I was also told, I that I was one of the patients' hospital personnel watched with great interest. They had observed the condition I was in when I first arrived and they watched my progress with a lot of interest. It seemed the whole hospital was watching my recovery progress. Many times they told me I was a miracle.

Each hospital visit I made they took as many as twenty x-rays; I probably should glow in the dark. I had crushed the bones in my lower left leg just above the ankle, and the bones in my upper left leg just above the knee. I totally blew out my left elbow, broke two fingers, both wrists and the bones in my upper left arm above the elbow. The problems were how to grow new tissue where there wasn't any tissue without removing my left leg. Like I said in the preface, Dr. Ebraheim said he was a *fighter* and that was exactly what he did. Praise God.

At first, my left leg and foot were turned in as if I was pigeon toed. During several of the operations they manipulated my leg--straightening my foot and knee. Actually, I believe they had to reform my foot. I was never informed if I had broken my left foot; however, it is a lot wider than my right foot and one inch shorter. The knuckle at the big toe is fixed so it doesn't bend, and it is thicker than my right big toe. That big toe being fixed makes it difficult going up and down stairs. My left ankle is fixed too in a right angle position. If I stand on it or have it flat on the floor, I can push my foot down and raise myself up and down. Somehow, it stays at the right angle, and I don't need a brace to walk. It is quite surprising how much you need your feet to be the same length and your toes to be mobile. Keeping your balance is quite difficult and I never realized that before.

Early on while I was still at Parkside, a pin in my left knee was protruding out into the skin, like a finger being poked into the tight skin of a blown up balloon. The pin had to be removed to prevent it from breaking through the skin.

A plastic surgeon from the hospital was called in to look at my injuries. She was asked to give her opinion on how she would close my open wounds. She operated manipulating the muscles and tissues around on my left arm to cover the open hole on my elbow. This procedure was done more than once and over time, with the help of a wound vac, that hole did close. To this day it is tender; but, the bone is covered. My elbow is also in a fixed position-maybe a thirty degree angle-perfect for carrying a purse on my left shoulder and resting my hand on it. I am unable to turn my left hand over; and, my arm is about four inches shorter than my right. My little finger and my ring finger do not bend like the others and I am unable to make a closed fist. In the beginning, I couldn't touch my thumb to any of my other fingers, but with therapy they now work very well-not perfect-but certainly well enough.

One of the next surgeries was my left lower leg. There was so much damage the wound vac wasn't working. The plastic surgeon had another idea which we ran with. In a twelve hour operation, she took a muscle from my stomach, attached the blood vessels from my ankle to the muscle, laid it over the open wound on my leg and covered it with skin graphed my right upper leg. That was called a *muscle flap*.

Prior to this operation, an arteriogram had to be done, making sure I had working veins in my ankle. I was laying on a gurney in the hallway waiting to go into the room for the test and a technician came out to tell me about the procedure. I was good until she said, "we use iodine dye". I am so allergic to iodine dye! Even though, they assured and reassured me many times over that everything would be alright, I would not let them take me into that room for an arteriogram! A young intern was called to talk to me about the procedure because the ladies were not convincing me. He told me how I was a miracle and that they would not let anything happen to me; that I had come so far since entering the hospital…. I started crying. I told him I was scared because of my allergy to the dye. I can't tell you how many times that young man said, "You are a miracle. W e are not going to let anything happen to you." I think if he could've picked me up and held me in his arms--he would have. He didn't, but, I could feel his compassion. It was probably forty-five minutes later when I gave in and let them do the test. I was scared, but the technicians and the doctor were good.

Following the operations I was put in the cardiac care unit because of overcrowding on the other floors. The nurses were supposed to keep a constant vigil for a pulse in the newly attached muscle. Plus, the doctor ordered that my room stay at a steady temperature of 85 degrees with a warming blanket over my leg. The first set of nurses was wonderful-they followed the doctor's instructions. The second set of nurses thought they would do their own thing. I woke up chilled; someone had turned the heat down and when I questioned the temperature in my room, they claimed the thermostat wouldn't go up to 85 degrees. Plus, they were not checking the *muscle flap* in the right location to hear the pulse. I was boiling!!! I knew they thought I was just being a pain and a complainer, but, I wasn't. I was scared. I'd just been through a twelve hour surgery, and it was my leg they were messing with! The doctor was even worried about the flap possibly dying, because she had such a terrible time connecting the blood vessels-they kept collapsing. At one point, she left the surgery room to tell Wayne she had tried to connect the blood vessels twice and failed. She was going to try one more time and if that didn't work they would have to come up with another solution. Consequently, she had been adamant about the kind of care I was to get before she left that night. The next day, when the doctor came in, I told her what had happened the night before and I believe she took care of the problem. I think the nurses were not happy that I was in their unit-they were very nasty. The next day I was moved to a step-down floor to be observed for at least a week. After the week, the flap seemed to be pulsating and going well so I went back to Parkside. What a relief!

At Parkside I was set up with a pull-up trapeze bar and they tied my leg up so it was even with my body. The doctor wanted the blood flowing evenly to the flap. She didn't want my leg lying on the bed because then it would be at a lower elevation than my heart nor did she want it at a higher elevation-that would restrict the blood flow to the flap. My leg certainly was not pretty; but, it was there, for now anyway! At this point, I can't tell you how many surgeries I had been through. I know there had been many. At this point, there were three plates in my lower left leg, with an external fixator attached to the leg, pins in both knees, a rod in my left upper leg, pins in the two fingers on my left hand, pins in both wrists, two screws in my left elbow, and two plates and screws in my upper left arm. My stomach had been opened up twice; once to remove my spleen and once to remove a muscle. I now have a five pack instead of a six pack.

Following my last surgery, I had been diagnosed with MRSA (staph infection) due to cross contamination of a skin graft. The skin used for the graft was transferred from my right leg over to my left. MRSA could have been fatal if they had not treated it properly. While at the hospital, I was quarantined. People could visit, but, they could not touch me or anything I had touched. They had to wear gloves and a gown, and change everything each time they came and went from my room. At least that was how it worked at the hospital. At Parkside they didn't care-according to them, everyone had MRSA. I did convince some of the aides to put on gloves. *Okay! What's next?*

Chapter VIIII

It was a pretty sunny morning and I thought I'd call Aprell. We were talking and, for some reason, I had trouble pronouncing my words. My tongue seemed to be swollen, and my mouth was dry. *Maybe I'm having some kind of an allergic reaction to my meds.* We talked for a minute; but, I was also talking to people in my room that were not actually in my room. Aprell wanted to know what was going on. I didn't know what to tell her so I hung up the phone and called the nurse. I don't remember what the nurse said and the time lapse escapes me; but, I remember talking to the ladies that change my wound vacs and bandages. Their demeanors were standoffish and aloof and I couldn't figure that out. One lady said they couldn't change my bandages because of some sort of complaint they had received. Then they left my room. The next thing I remembered was; I had to go to the bathroom and I had a hard time getting someone to help me. When someone finally came to put a bed pan under me, they didn't come back to take it out from under me. After waiting for what seemed an hour, I took it out myself; at least, I thought I did. I remember thrashing around in the bed something terrible. I couldn't keep still. My muscles were jumping and twitching. A housekeeping lady came into my room and asked me what was wrong. I told her I didn't know what was wrong and I couldn't get anyone to answer my call. She said she would go find someone because what I was doing was not good. When she returned, she said she had been told I had to work through whatever it was I was going through. I rolled over and said "okay". I can't tell you how long I thrashed about in that bed-it seemed like a very long time.

In the evening I physically calmed down some, but, my mind was going full blast. I remember thinking I was in some kind of sleeping pod-again with no floor-just a narrow ledge and a hammock type bed that went from one end to the other. Wayne was sleeping in a hammock bed next to mine. I was afraid I would fall and Wayne was angry with me because I wouldn't get in the hammock and go to sleep. He couldn't see what I was seeing. I finally got into the bed and tried to go to sleep; but, I was worried. I thought we were in a futuristic concentration camp. The next thing I remember is running away. Wayne was pushing me down the road on a gurney and we are trying to hide from the nurses and aides at the home. We came into Monroe and were hiding in a classroom at our church school. When school opened in the morning, we had to leave. We went to our actual home. Wayne pushed me into the garage and came right back out. I was standing outside the garage door in a square box. I looked down and the sidewalk disappeared out from under me and I found myself standing on another narrow ledge at the top of a deep dark shaft. I thought Wayne left me to fend for myself. Eventually, he came back to get me and we were back at Parkside. Wayne asked me what was wrong and why was I acting so strangely. I didn't know why. I didn't realize I was acting any different than usual. He wouldn't listen to me or I couldn't get across to him what was going on in my head. He was frustrated and I gave up trying to convey my concerns to him.

Later on, while I was lying in my bed at the nursing home, I looked up at the swinging triangle above my head and panic gripped me! *The triangle! The sign of Satan!* Then, out of nowhere, there was a young boy standing in front of me up by the triangle. This boy's complexion was pale- almost an ash grey: he had short curly light brown hair, was slight in build and looked more like an image of a person, rather than an actual person. He stood there looking at me. I asked him his name- he did not respond. I asked him if Satan had sent him, and he nodded his head *yes*. I asked him if he had come for me and he nodded *yes* again. I tried to reason with him…to no avail…so I told him to go away; which, he did for now. My heart was pumping!

The nurse didn't like the way I was acting so I was sent to the hospital; only to return in the same state I left in. I was talking to the other person in the bed next to mine; I told that person I was going to die. That the nurses and aides were practicing Satanism and I was going to be their human sacrifice. I said I had seen a gang murder on TV and the body was dumped into a big garbage dumpster and that was what was going to happen to me. I thought the people in the nursing home were in a conspiracy, they were plotting to sacrifice someone, and that someone was going to be me. I began screaming for help trying to find someone who would listen to me and help me. The boy appeared above me again, motioning for me to follow him. This time a woman was with the boy. She was standing at the head of my bed. She was an older black woman, short in stature, chubby, straight hair down to her shoulders. I thought she was coaching the young boy how to convince me to follow them. I yelled for them to leave me alone! I wasn't going to follow the Devil! No matter what! They left again. The male nurse came in and gave me a shot to calm me down. Apparently, I was getting way to loud and making accusations of Devil worshipping. He did not like my accusations. I apologized; but, that was what I saw and it was *very* real to me. The hallucinations didn't stop there. They got scarier and I was gripped with heart stopping fear.

I observed a commune of some sort back in the woods. There were a lot of people milling around setting up for a ritual celebration. The male nurse, his wife, and family were there. It seemed to me, they were getting ready for the celebration too. The male nurse had a little girl around the age of two. She was the center of everyone's attention. I watched through the bushes and trees with apprehension. I wanted to see what is going on or what was going to happen. There was a rustic cabin, and a bon fire in an open area with tall pine trees all around. I spotted a concrete slab; four feet high, four feet wide, and six feet long with a big butcher knife lying on it. There were lit candles circling the slab. I saw people wearing long black capes with hoods walking around the circle chanting something I couldn't understand. The male nurse brought his little girl to a person standing at the concrete slab. I was horrified! My heart was pounding out of my chest! I ran out to the circle and screamed at him not to let them hurt her! *Doesn't he know what they are going to do? Where was his wife?* He walked over to me and said everything was okay and he left; leaving his little girl with these insane people. I panicked. I ran around desperately trying to convince someone to stop the insanity! Unfortunately, the little girl was sacrificed right in front of me! They removed her heart and held it up for everyone to see; her blood was running down the assassinator's arm! No one cared, they continued to chant and walk around the burning candles. I believed I was next. They grabbed me, took me into the cabin and began prepping me for sacrifice. I had to get away. I waited for the right moment and ran away as fast and as far as I could; but, I didn't know where I was or which was to run.

It was evening and getting dark. I saw dim lights in the distance. I had come across an isolated house in the woods. I approached with caution and looked inside through a window. The family came outside and embraced my presence as if I had been there all along. They had two teenage daughters, and their youngest daughter was to be sacrificed along with me. *Help! Get me out of here!* I looked up and there was a CNA standing beside me trying her best to calm me down and make sense of what I was telling her. I heard her rebuke the Devil out of my room. (I did not hallucinate that.) I heard her yell, "Devil! I rebuke you! Get out of this room!" I saw her right arm fling up and out ordering Satan to leave. I thanked her and asked her to do it again. She shook her head "No" and said she couldn't. I understood; the male nurse probably told her not to. I saw another CNA walk past the foot of my bed and as she did so she said, "This is Spiritual Warfare, that's what this is."

My husband was called to come to the nursing home. He didn't know what to think. He couldn't understand what was happening to me or why. I tried to talk to him and tell him what I thought was going on. And, at the same time, I was afraid of someone overhearing me tell Wayne my thoughts. I was *petrified* that the Devil was trying to kill me and take my soul. I tried to tell Wayne not to leave me because the Devil was after me. I thought, if he left, they would appear to put something in my IV that would make my heart stop beating. In fact, the two individuals were there, but, Wayne couldn't see them or hear what I thought they were saying. I prayed to God to make these two people go away. They were so real; I actually thought I was going to die.

I was sent to the hospital a second time; and again, they checked me over and I was found to be in good physical condition. Everyone thought I was going crazy. I was left alone in a room waiting for the EMTS to arrive. I clung to the Bible that I held in my hands and I talked to a doctor e for a bit. We talked about the Bible and I asked him if he went to church and what his favorite verse was. He obliged by telling me. He wrote it down on a piece of paper and signed his name to it. After the doctor left, the demons returned. I was getting so worn down fighting against them. I felt I should give up. I opened the Bible and began reading. Up over my head and behind me was an invisible demon. It began spraying a liquid mist over the top of me. The mist was falling down on me and the pages of the Bible, washing the words off the pages as I read. For some reason I thought it was an acid wash and I thought I had been defeated.

The ambulance arrived to take me back to Parkside. The trip seemed awfully long and the driver was driving fast and reckless. I wondered *how could I be sure they were taking me where they were supposed to take me?* I almost panicked. Then I maintained my composure and decided to lie still. I tried to stay calm, even though my heart was pumping overtime. Needless to say, I was confused and scared to death.

I arrived at Parkside at 4:00 a.m. The nurse took my blood pressure which was very low. I don't remember what the reading was; but, I do remember that it was low enough that I wanted the nurse to call a doctor. She said she couldn't disturb the doctor at that time in the morning and I had to wait until 7:30 a.m. She said my blood pressure wasn't bad. The bottom number was around 43 which is really low. She continued to tell me she wasn't worried about the bottom number. The top one was the number she would be concerned with. I told her I knew better than that and I would die if she didn't call a doctor. I argued; but, she walked out on me. In her haste, she didn't put my leg up in the sling. I was positioned at the foot of the bed; and, I felt myself slipping off the end of the bed. There wasn't a floor underneath the end of the bed, just another bottomless pit. I wriggled until I got myself up to the head of the bed where I could reach the telephone and I called the police. However, I didn't know the address of Parkside, so that didn't work.

I forced down some dry bread and thick, sticky peanut butter in an attempt to raise my blood pressure-and I waited-determined not to let them kill me. Eventually, the nurse came back, discovered she didn't put my leg up and, by this time, the flap was bleeding all over the bed. She called for help to raise my leg and put a clean bandage on it.

About 6:30 a.m. the head nurse came in to check on me. We talked for a few minutes then she said she decided to call the ambulance and Wayne. I thanked her very much. I was so scared. In fact, I was terrified!

The EMTS people came into my room, asked me what was going on, I started crying and said, "I think they're trying to kill me." These EMTs had transported me many times before, they knew me, and they looked very concerned. They told me to take it easy; they would take me out of there immediately. When I was put in the ambulance, the paramedic began strapping me in; but, before he could do that he wanted to set my Bible aside. I started struggling with him. *He was not taking my Bible!* I felt the Bible was the only thing keeping me from being taken by the Devil and I wasn't giving it up! The paramedic talked to me and was looking at me strangely. He couldn't understand what was going on. I, finally, gave the Bible up to him. I asked him to read to me until we got to the hospital. He did the best he could without his glasses.

I was taken into the emergency room where Wayne was waiting. Aprell came in a little while later, followed by the doctor. The paramedic that read to me told the doctor that something was seriously wrong. He said they had transported me many times before and I was not acting like the same women they knew.

Prior to arriving at the hospital, Aprell made a detour. She went to Parkside and asked the nurse to open the med book for her to look at. As she suspected, I had been taking oxycotin for pain-30 milligrams twice a day. Somehow, someone cut me off of the oxy *cold turkey.* Oxycotin is a narcotic that a patient should be weaned off from, not abruptly stopped. That threw me into withdrawals. That weekend was my worst nightmare. My plastic surgeon, said no one had permission to stop the oxycotin. She immediately put me back on it and I was admitted into the hospital. Wayne called the State to investigate Parkside; but, of course, everything was found to be in compliance with State laws. Needless to say, I did not return to Parkside. In fact, our pastor from church went there to pick up my belongings. Wayne was too upset to go back.

I stayed in the hospital for a week. Aprell spent two nights with me. At night, I would fidget with my covers and talk to no one in the room until Aprell asked me what I was doing. Once the meds started working, I felt better. I wasn't hallucinating anymore. I was still pretty upset and very much afraid to be alone. I didn't know what would have happened without Wayne and Aprell. That weekend was extremely frightening for me and my family. I held onto my Bible because I thought it was my only lifeline; and, actually it was. Without my faith, I think I would have died from fear. The mind is an amazing part of the human body.

The hospital staff was trying so hard to work with me. I was so blessed. I talked to a nurse who asked me if I had ever read the book, "90 Minutes In Heaven" by Don Piper. I said I hadn't, so she wrote the title and author down for me encouraging me to read the book. Then she asked me if I had kept notes or a journal of the events that had been happening to me. Of course, I didn't. It's all engraved in my head. She also thought that I should write my own book. That thought never crossed my mind. Besides, I had been marking an X in place of my name for about three months. Keeping notes or a journal wasn't possible.

According to one intern, I had a very long road ahead of me; and, my recovery had only just begun. I didn't understand that the road was going to be as long as he had tried to get across to me. I didn't think my injuries were as serious as he knew they were. My lack of knowledge was a blessing. Praise God.

Chapter X

F ear gripped me at the thought of going back to Parkside; and, I had way too many things going on for Wayne to take me home. . Pastor made a couple of nursing home suggestions for Wayne to check out. This time he was making personal visits to the homes prior to my being moved anywhere. My guardian angels had been working overtime keeping me safe and I was sure this next place would be a good place. There were several nursing homes in the town we lived in; however, some of the clients from the Department of Corrections, Probation/Parole Office worked in those nursing homes prior to a law being passed that nursing home employees had to have background checks before being hired. Even though that law was in effect at the time of my accident, I did run into a previous client at Parkside. He wasn't working on the floor I was staying on; but, when he was called to help move a patient on another floor he complied. Just so happened, that patient ended up being me. He recognized me and I recognized him; but, that chance encounter convinced me even more that my coming to Monroe would not be a wise decision.

The middle of September, 2006 I was transported to Harbor Towne Care Center in Point Place, Ohio-just over the Michigan/Ohio border- only about fifteen minutes from home. Wayne visited this care center, told them everything I had going on and that I had been taking the antibiotic, Vancomycin, which was being used to combat the MRSA. The Vanco made me very sick to my stomach when it was administered prior to my eating. In order for me to keep food down, I needed to get the vanco after all meals. That was the order in which the hospital had been giving it to me. I was getting way to thin and not keeping food down, of course, didn't help. The plastic surgeon made it known that I needed to add some weight Wayne made arrangements with the supervisors at Harbor Towne that I would receive the vancomycin in the evening around 8:30 p.m. after all meals. Plus, our insurance case worker ordered me a private room due to all my open wounds. It seemed, we were all set and I was ready to be moved.

I arrived at Harbor Towne around 9:00 p.m. in the evening–too late. If we had known it was going to take that long to get me there, we would not have made the trip that evening. However, there was a welcoming committee waiting when we arrived. It was a middle-aged nurse with long blonde hair; short and slim in stature, friendly, very talkative, and nervous. Along with her was a man in a wheelchair about my age, 54. He was scruffy looking with longer dark brown curly hair, thinning on top. He was supporting an external fixator on his right leg due to a motorcycle accident. He introduced himself and gave us a short synopsis of why he was there. I'd guessed he thought we had something in common so he came out to greet us-which we appreciated. Him and Wayne stood in the hallway for a while and talked while the nurse settled me in.

My room was very nicely decorated, homey, and big in comparison to Parkside. The next day I was introduced to some of the CNAs who would be responsible for my care. I remembered them standing in the doorway looking at me with-don't know-apprehension. I thought I might be in trouble again. The lead nurse on the floor came in and introduced herself. She stated she was the one in charge, and everyone else had to do what she said. I had a feeling we were going to possibly have a problem-with an attitude like that; but, I give everyone the benefit of the doubt.

The first thing she did was order a trapeze from another home affiliated with this home for my leg-which was the right thing to do. When the trapeze arrived, she ordered weights be put on my left leg, which was the wrong thing to do, and she would *not* listen. Finally, Wayne told her to recheck the orders with the hospital. Our insurance case worker got involved too. By that evening, the weights came off and my leg was tied up evenly with my heart the way it was suppose to be. What a mess!

The second night this same lead nurse had been to an evening meeting, and she came in around 8:30 p.m. to administer my vancomycin, as arranged by Wayne prior to my arrival. That was good; things seemed to be going along okay. This lead nurse, I thought, was a nice person just insecure in her position. After everything I had just been through, though, I really didn't want to be used as a proving point to the rest of the staff for her.

The third or fourth day, the same lead nurse came into my room shaking her finger at me saying that from then on I would be getting my vancomycin first thing in the mornings rather than in the evenings. She said she didn't have any nurses on duty at night licensed to administer the medicine. I tried to tell her the medicine made me sick to my stomach. I couldn't keep food down after taking it, and I couldn't afford to lose any more weight. The doctors were telling me to gain weight; plus, it had been prearranged that I get the medicine after all my meals. I only had two weeks left to take the vancomycin. She did not care; she said it was what it was and I would get the medicine in the mornings. I felt exceptionally vulnerable and not in a state of mind to argue with her. I started crying. The floor nurse came in, busied herself with my bandages, and said, "Go over her head. As a patient you have rights. She is overstepping her bounds. Go to your Patient Advocate." I called Wayne almost immediately; he was my Patient Advocate. That night, a nurse who usually worked evenings on the nursing home side of Harbor Towne, came into my room to administer the vancomycin. She said she just lived down the road and would come in and give me the medicine until it was done. It wasn't a big deal for her. I couldn't thank her enough. Praise God. He had my best interest in mind.

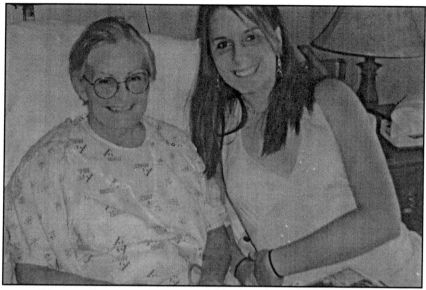

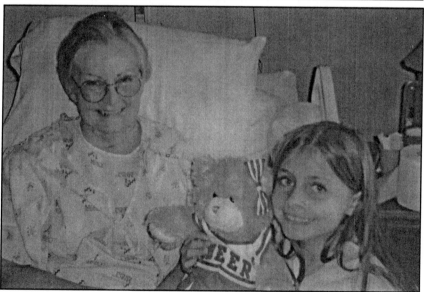

Brittany & Brandi Visiting

After all the bumps in the road, some members of our contemporary church band came to my room and sang some songs. It was wonderful! Wayne and I cried. They made us feel like we weren't going through all of this totally alone and forgotten. Their visit was truly uplifting. They returned to the nursing home at a later date and sang for all the residents. I felt very blessed to have them come and sing for us. It was an enlightening time in the midst of, what was a pretty depressing place.

It didn't take long before the therapy team came around trying to get me up and about. I remember a therapist getting me into a wheelchair: pulling along my IV pole, holding both my wound vac machines, and pushing me down the perfectly polished hallway to get a look at where I lived. We went a little too far though-the therapist got tired. My equipment was too heavy for the little therapist and we had to return to my room. It was a nice adventure though. I enjoyed it. She gave me the feeling that I was getting better and a little stronger. I wasn't as strong as I thought, though, and I was still bed bound. Every time I would dangle my left leg over the edge of the bed blood would drip onto the floor and I would have to put my leg back up. The muscle flap on my leg didn't want to heal completely closed; consequently I made many trips to the hospital for operations to debriede the flap. It would be opened, flushed out then sewed closed. I couldn't tell you how many times that procedure was done, it was many. All in all, over the four year period, I had endured forty-two operations total.

I tried to be uplifting and keep my depression under wraps. At times, it was very difficult to have a positive attitude. After the medicine incident, the lead nurse pretty much ignored me and Wayne-which was okay. Everyone else seemed to be doing the best they knew how to take care of me. And, when I stop to think about it, I was a lot of work for the CNAs. For about the first three to five months, all of my hygiene was done while I was in bed. Later on, I became more mobile. I could get out of bed, but, the CNAs had to lift me. They had to lift me in the bathroom, showers, chairs, etc. Not to mention, with each visit to the hospital, my orders changed. I could put full weight on my legs, then partial weight, and at other times no weight at all. I would take two steps forward and one back.

The CNAs had different procedures that I had to get used to. They wanted to know every teeny tiny personal activity that I did. To put my bra on, one CNA would tell me to put the boulders in their sling holders; another one called them the *girls*. I was allowed only one bath per week which I definitely was not used to. I was told to use one wash cloth for the top and another one for the bottom. Who uses two wash cloths to take a shower? And, when they dried me, they would get in between each of my toes. My left leg had to be wrapped in a clear plastic bag that was taped to my skin so the water would not penetrate it. We didn't know at first if the fixator could get wet or not.

A couple two or three weeks into my stay at Harbor Towne a young man arrived to live there. He was put in the room across the hall from me. He had been a patient there before and was on a return trip due to diabetes, drug usage, and unable to take care of himself. However, he did get around pretty well in his wheelchair; and, there was more to his story than I was told or wanted to know. Not long after his arrival the little blonde nurse came to me and said I was going to be moved to the other end of the building away from this young man. I didn't know if she had something to do with my being moved or not. She did say she knew him and didn't want me down at that end of the hallway with him across the hall. The nurse's station was too far away. I was okay with the move as long as I wasn't right at the nurse's station. That area was always busy and noisy.

Eventually, I was moved into a room at the other end of the building. It wasn't quite as homey as the one I left; but, I had a better view outside the window. I could see the bay from this room, some scenery and; once in a while, an animal. All the rooms shared bathrooms with the room next door. In the beginning my neighbors were two elderly ladies; one was bedridden and pretty much nonresponsive. The other lady walked around using a walker and, I thought, she had it pretty much mentally together.

There were two men in one room down the hall that were living in the home mainly because they were homeless. I don't know for sure how they came to get into the home in the first place; but, they must have had something medically wrong. And, once they were patients, the home couldn't make them leave-because they didn't have anywhere to go. I understood that they had been there for quite some time.

Another man living at Harbor Towne was an amputee. He had lost a leg due to diabetes; and, was living at the nursing home due to an infection. He had actually been there in the past for similar problems. He pretty much kept to himself. I don't remember him receiving any visitors either.

A couple ladies I met were permanently living on the rehab side of the building because they wanted to be with people who were more alert than the nursing home side residents. I enjoyed their company throughout my stay which ended up being ten months. This was definitely an environment I had never encountered before. I had visited Wayne's grandmother in the nursing home before; but, that was a whole different ball game.

The reality of being in a nursing home/rehab facility hit me hard when the bedridden, nonresponsive lady next door died. Then her roommate came down with pneumonia. I overheard my *favorite* head nurse ask this little old frail lady if she wanted the staff to resuscitate her in the event that her heart would stop. The nurse said, "If I have to do CPR on you, I will break your chest bones. Is that what you want me to do?" Of course, the little old lady said, "No, just let me go." Needless to say, I did not like that conversation at all. It was a true statement; but, the nurse was too blunt and cold.

I pretty much lost it one evening after that just before Wayne left for the day. My world came crashing down around my shoulders, my legs were spasming, and I was crying hysterically. The floor nurse and Wayne were about to pull their hair out-Wayne didn't have that much hair to lose. The nurse gave me all the medicine I was allowed to take but, it took a while before it finally took hold-otherwise, I was going to the hospital. Having been that close to death and knowing others were dying just on the other side of the wall, brought me face to face with the reality of my situation. I didn't come to this facility to die; at least, I hoped I didn't. To make matters worse, I was still battling MRSA (staph infection) and an older, black, female CNA told me that her mother came to this same nursing home with MRSA and died before they could get it under control. That certainly did not help my mental state!

After getting some of my frustrations out of my system, I began to settle into my new, I hoped-temporary home. I still had to get used to the CNAs and they had to get used to me. For the most part, everyone was very nice and treated me well. I thought I was making quite a few friends throughout my stay at Harbor Towne. I learned at lot from some of the ladies. I also learned later on that, when I first arrived, most of the personnel were afraid to work with me because of Wayne-my Patient Advocate. Our reputation had preceded us and that wasn't a bad thing either. Not to mention, they weren't used to someone with as many injuries as I had. The other injured motorcyclist had similar injuries; but, I believe mine were somewhat more extensive. We were both blessed to be alive. After everyone got to know Wayne and me, they relaxed and acted normal. They would come into my room and tell us their personal problems or the problems they had at the home. Sometimes I felt like their mother or their best friend. I did a lot of listening and that was a good thing. Listening took my mind off of myself.

My co-workers took up donations and got me a VCR and some tapes to watch while I was bed-ridden. I was so surprised and happy to have them do something that nice for me. The only problem I had was being confined to my bed, and I couldn't get the tapes in or out of the VCR. I had to wait for Wayne to visit then we would watch the movies together. We were introduced to a Tyler Perry movie which was so funny. We had never heard of him before; but, we really enjoyed watching that movie.

While at Harbor Towne, I received some beautiful flowers from my Prayer Partner. The flowers were so full of pretty cheerful colors. I didn't realize I had a prayer partner, or who that person might have been. I wanted to thank them for the flowers and the prayers. I appreciated both.

One of our friends from church came to visit a few times. Every time she came she would massage my feet, put lotion on them, and clean them up for me. My feet would get dry and flakey so her rubbing them felt good. I loved her taking the time to visit and actually wanting to massage my feet. The CNAs would wash them, but, our lady friend massaged and put lotion on them. Oh, I almost forgot. Around Christmas time a nurse decided to put nail polish on my toes. She thought they should be dressed up for the holidays. She was funny. Wayne came in and said, "What is *that* on your toes?" We all got a good laugh out of his response.

I had to do both physical therapy and occupational therapy which was a good thing. It was very slow at first. Physical therapy was responsible for getting me up and out of bed and into a wheelchair; which was what was coming along slow. They also had me doing range of motion exercises, walking a little with a walker or the parallel bars depending on how much weight I was allowed to put on my legs, and what I had just had operated on, which changed every week or two. I had so many objects attached to me getting around was hard.

Occupational therapy would come into my room in the mornings to help me bathe myself, brush my teeth, and do general every day morning grooming. I must admit it was difficult because I used to be a left handed person. Since I had limited use of my left hand and arm, doing every day things the normal way for me had changed. I mentioned earlier eating with my right hand when I used to use my left all the time. There were other changes too. For instance, combing my hair, I could not reach my head with my left hand. Putting make-up on-Prior to the accident, I used my right arm/hand for my right side and my left arm/hand for my left side. Putting pierced earrings in both ears with one hand, hooking a necklace with one hand, buttoning jeans or a blouse with one hand was a learning experience. All these things I took for granted when I was *normal*.

One morning, I remember a therapist asked me if I would like to get dressed and out of the hospital gowns I had been wearing for about four or five months. I was so surprised, I questioned, Can I?" *What a novel idea!* The thought of putting on real clothes was wonderful! One problem, I didn't have any of my own clothes at the nursing home. And, what was I going to get over the external fixator on my leg. Wayne had to bring me in some tee-shirts and a couple pair of *his* shorts. He also went to the Bali store and got me some underwear. You know the commercials where the lady asks, "What size is she" and the guy says "About your size"? That was exactly what Wayne did. I got a kick out of that. At first, I thought he might have been a little embarrassed; but, then I thought, it was Wayne. He wouldn't be embarrassed The nursing home was pretty warm all year long so the shorts and tees were perfect. Wayne's shorts were big enough through the legs to go over the fixator-they looked like skorts on me. They were perfect. I thought I was making a lot of progress by actually putting on regular clothes. What a great feeling!

Chapter XI

After the two ladies next door passed away, my next neighbors were two men; a black man and a Pollock. The black man was hard of hearing and every time he spoke he yelled. He didn't speak with me at all; but, I could hear everything he said to everybody else no matter where he was on that wing of the building. The Pollock was in his late eighties. He was attractive for his age, tall with silver hair and friendly. He was at the nursing home for rehab after a knee replacement. At first, he would come knocking on my door to visit with me and Wayne. Later on, he would wait for Wayne to leave *then* he would come visit me. His name was Staush. He told me all about his wife and child, who were not alive; and, his girlfriend, who was ninety plus years old and lived next door to his home. He loved her so much, but he felt her son did not want them together. I was sad for him. He brought her to my room once so I could meet with her. She was well kept and attractive. I could see why Staush was so excited to have her in his life.

Staush educated me on how the Polish people came to Toledo, Ohio. He even tried to teach me how to speak Polish, which was hilarious. The CNAs and nurses would walk past my room, peek in and gesture with their hands like a telephone asking, "Do you want me to call you?" because his visits would take quite awhile. One day Staush brought his nephew and wife into therapy to meet me. I was surprised.. The therapists asked me if we were related and I told them no we were just friends. He was cute though, he took it upon himself to be my bodyguard. I didn't know him before he came to Harbor Towne. Wayne jokingly said he was going to have to put my wedding ring back on my finger. Staush ended up going to live with his nephew and family; and, that made him feel down because he didn't think he could continue to see his girlfriend anymore.

People came and went often from Harbor Towne. I made friends with a ninety year old lady in a wheelchair that would sit at the front of the building looking out the large windows almost every day. She had one daughter who would come visit her once in a while. The daughter wasn't there as often as the elderly lady would have liked; and, I felt sorry for her. She was sad and depressed. I attempted to cheer her up. I would meet her at the windows in the mornings, and we would talk. One morning she said the room just around the corner had been raided by the police the night before. Surprised I exclaimed, "What?" She shook her head, *yup*. She said men in suits and uniforms went into the room; shut the door and pretty much turned the room upside down. Then she said she heard the patient in that room told that he had to appear in Court sometime in the future. He wasn't arrested because he had a car accident, broke his leg and was in the home for therapy. I had heard about drugs floating around between some of the patients who lived down that hall; but, this little old lady's story sure did surprise me.

Some of the patients, like the motorcycle accident guy and the young man in the wheelchair with diabetes, were drug users prior to arriving at the nursing home. There was a young woman with some kind of muscle problem admitted to the home for therapy who was also involved with the drug usage. She would leave home in the afternoon following therapy; then in the evening either high or drunk. All three of those patients somehow would get drugs into the nursing home. I was *flabbergasted* with everything that was going on. The nurses would have fits because they couldn't dispense medicine to those people when they were high or had been drinking; and, the patients couldn't be stopped from leaving the home as long as they were back the same day. Then, when the patients wouldn't get their meds, they would get upset and call for investigation of the nursing home for improper practices. This was ongoing.

The motorcycle guy told me about an incident where he got into a shouting match with his roommate over music or the TV being too loud. His roommate picked up a radio and threw it at him; in turn, he grabbed his IV monitor to throw it at back his roommate when the nurse came into the room. Then police were called to the nursing home. Maybe that was part of what my little old lady friend heard and saw. After all that the motorcycle guy wanted to leave the home *right now*.

At about 1:00 a.m. in the morning I was awake and reading, when I heard a soft knock on my door, and a male's voice requesting to come in. It was the motorcycle guy. I couldn't imagine what he wanted that time of the morning. He asked we could talk for a minute. I said we could talk for a little while. I had no idea what he could possibly want to talk about. He wheeled over to my bed and said, "I'm having a real hard time." His injuries were taking forever to heal, he was in pain, and, emotionally, the setbacks were getting to him. He looked at me and said, "How do you do it?" I looked at him--puzzled. .He repeated himself, "How do you do it? You seem to be so calm and in good spirits all the time. It doesn't seem to be bothering you to be in here like it is me." I wasn't so sure I agreed with his observations; but, there just happened to be a "Portals of Prayer" devotion booklet lying on the table in front of me and I took that moment to witness to this guy. I said, "I pray, read my devotions and the Bible passages; they calm me, give me hope, patience and strength." He thanked me and said, "good night". I sat there wondering if I had said enough or if I had said what he needed-I wasn't skilled at witnessing.

This guy's son lived in Florida and wanted our doctor to transfer his case down there He was going through some of the same set backs as I was with our lower legs. I didn't think Dr. Ebraheim would transfer him; but, he left the nursing home and moved to Florida anyway. Probably a month later, Wayne and I saw him at the hospital following his move. He was on crutches and moved along fairly well-still not putting pressure on his leg. He had returned from Florida for an appointment with the doctor. We never saw him again after that.

The little man across the hall and north of me a few doors came into my room one evening to introduce himself to me. He seemed like a good man just not healthy in mind or body. He was one of the men that came into the nursing home because of his diabetes and never left due to being homeless. Anyway, before he went back to his room, he invited me for a beer. I told him, "Thank you, but, no thank you". I was shocked! I wasn't aware nursing homes allowed beer on the premises let alone in an individual's room. I talked to the nurse on duty informing her of the alcohol smell on my neighbor's breath. She confirmed he was an alcoholic along with being diabetic. She also advised me that a patient's room was considered their home and they were allowed to bring in whatever they wanted-including booze. I couldn't believe what I heard.

The big guy that shared the same room with the little man was also an alcoholic. I had no idea why he was living in the nursing home other than being homeless. This man made jewelry out of wire which he sold from somewhere. He had a car and would leave every day in the morning and return in the evening. Usually, the little man went with him. Most of the time they would return- looped. They would eat dinner and retire to their room until morning.

They always had a conflict with the nurses because, of course, medicine. Eventually, the jewelry maker did leave. I thought he actually ended up getting an apartment of his own. The little man kept drinking, going into the hospital, returning, and drinking some more. He was asked to leave the home due to his noncompliance with the rules or the nurses. He was so pathetic; it was as if he had a death wish.

He finally left the nursing home and when his room was cleaned out; needles were found hidden in his closet. He had been medicating himself. To me this was unreal! Probably a month later, we heard that he had died. The news of the little man's death upset some nurses and CNAs. They thought he had been kicked out wrongly; and, if he had stayed in the nursing home, he would not have died. I wasn't sure I agreed with their thoughts, especially watching the road he was going down. He and his partner shared a bathroom with two ladies, just like I shared a bathroom with two men. One night he came in drunk, went into the bathroom when his neighbor lady was in there sitting on the pot. He gave her a big kiss on the lips! She screamed bringing everyone to the bathroom. The poor lady was in shock, and her family was even more upset. The next day room changes began. Two women were moved in next door to me to share my bathroom. The men got two men as neighbors to share their bathroom. I thought at the time that bathroom sharing should be women with women and men with men.

There was an older lady staying at the home following the amputation of her leg. She had returned to Harbor Towne because of diabetes, infection and the removal of her leg. Unfortunately, she had gotten to the point of wanting her leg removed. She said she was tired of being in rehab and continually fighting infections. She wanted to go home and stay there. She did not like living in the nursing home and she made her feelings known. She was an unhappy lady; but not quite ready for Harbor Towne to become her permanent home.

A couple that was living in the nursing home wanted to be married to each other. They were probably in their fifties or thereabouts. She had MS and was confined to a wheelchair. I wasn't sure what was going on with the man; but, they wanted to be married-they were both permanent residents in the home. She would get mad at her fiancée, cuss him up one side and down the other and throw things at him! But, she insisted she loved him and kept asking if they could be married. Wayne and I asked if a wedding between two residents would be possible in a home like that. We were told if their families didn't object it could happen. I didn't know about that!

A fairly young man, probably in his forties, was living at the nursing home because of his MS. I don't know how long he had been a resident, but, he was alone. No one ever came to visit him. He had been married and did have two children now in his wife's custody. He was pretty mobile with a wheelchair so he was given a motorized chair to get around in. One day, I noticed, he was in his motorized chair and the next day he was in his manual chair. I asked him what happened, and he said, "They took it away from me…I was speeding down the hallways", he laughed and so did I. It was funny!

Wayne was leaving after a day long visit, and I went with him to the door. When I turned around to go back to my room, the young man was sitting in the hallway watching us. He asked, "Is that your husband?" I answered that he was. He said, "He stayed with you through all you've been through?" I said, "Yes". He said, "That's good my wife didn't." I felt terrible for him. I didn't know what to say other than I was sorry. He carried pictures of his kids and showed them to everyone. Before I was released from the nursing home, I heard his ex-wife finally brought his daughters to visit with him. It was still a sad case. Thank the Lord my husband did not listen to a friend of his and honored our marriage vows--*through sickness and health.*

There were a mother and daughter who shared a room down the hall from me. I didn't see the mother much; but, the daughter was out and about often. The mother was living there due to getting old and not being able to take care of herself. The daughter was living with her because she was mentally and physically handicapped. Apparently, there wasn't family to take care of them both. Suddenly, one day, the mom died. I wasn't sure if the daughter actually understood what had happened; but, she did realize that mom wasn't there anymore. It wasn't long before the daughter went into the hospital for some reason. Unfortunately, upon returning to the home, she passed away too. They had both been residents there for quite some time.

Grandma lived down the hallway from me on the same side. She was quite the character-over ninety years old. She never said much of anything to anyone. She just tooled around in her wheelchair going in and out of everyone's room. She would go through drawers and closets and when something that caught her eye, she took it with her. She came into my room once. I tried to talk to her. She stopped, looked at me for a few minutes, muttered something, turned around and left. I had no idea what was going through her head she never said a word. I was told her family was in Arizona. The family wanted to take her out there with them; but, she didn't want to go. She liked Harbor Towne and thought the people there liked her better than her family liked her. She was cherished by the nurses and aides. However, she kept them busy keeping her busy. Her family seemed to be waiting for her to die; they were impatient with her. She wasn't treated that way at the nursing home. Grandma was happy there.

We also had a retired priest stay with us for a while. He was a trip. He was arrogant and nasty to the nurses and aides. He wanted everything done his way or no way-even his treatment. He claimed he had heart problems, maybe he did, I didn't know for sure. At one point, he got upset because the nurses would not listen to him. He thought he knew better how they should take care of him. He called someone to take him out of the nursing home, and, they did--only to return at a later date. Unfortunately, when he came back, he met his match with his next roommate was Mr. Mott (fictitious name). I knew of Mr. Mott. He was from the Monroe area. His son had reported to our office for a while. Mr. Mott and his son had quite the reputation for being *nutty*.

One morning the priest was arguing with the aides, belittling them, swearing at them and calling them names. Mr. Mott stepped up to defend the girls and threatened to clobber the priest with his crutch. He told the priest he wouldn't stand for him treating the girls like that. He continued to tell the priest what he thought of him, his mouth, and his actions. The nurses ran into the room breaking up the fight before someone got hurt. Needless to say, the priest was moved to a new room and he actually had an attitude change.

For some reason, Mr. Mott took a liking to me. If he was at one end of the hallway and I was at the other end, he would yell at the top of his voice "Sandra!" He would come to my room and spend hours telling me all his problems with Monroe County's Sheriff's Department, his family and neighbors. Again, either a nurse or an aide would come to my door; put their fingers up as if they were talking on a telephone, motioning to me, did I want them to call me so he would leave. He would come to my room, knock on the door with his crutch and ask if I was okay. The nurses tried to steer him away, but he got upset with them. He was just checking on me and he wasn't going to stay!

Mr. Mott played musical instruments too. I believe one was a mandolin, and the other was the harmonica. He was actually pretty good too. He was taping music for different people that he liked at the nursing home. I think I was on his gift list; but, I left to go home before he got the tape finished. He got in his head that Wayne and I should renew our wedding vows, and he wanted to attend the service. Oh my gosh, he would see Wayne come into the building and follow him all the way down each hall talking to him about renewing our vows. This went on for at least two or three months. Mr. Mott even went so far as to ask the priest, he just about clobbered, to do the honors. We said we were not Catholic, but, that didn't matter to him. We were going to do what he wanted no matter what. When I left the home, his eyes filled with tears and he said, "If I were a younger man..." I took his picture and gave him a hug. He was a little mixed up in the head, but a dear old soul.

About the time Mr. Mott arrived at Harbor Towne a young woman with a broken leg also arrived. Her room was down the hall and across from the nurse's station. She was short, small in stature, had dark brown, straight hair a little longer than shoulder length-always wore it in a pony tail. She was plain but nice looking. She was very friendly; however, she had many physical problems. She came to the nursing/rehab home this time to recuperate from her broken leg which happened when she fell at home. I believe she tripped over a throw rug in her kitchen. Her first visit was the year before when she broke her back. I don't know how that happened. This young lady was thirty-two years old: suffering from heart problems, osteoporosis, and kidney failure. She would leave three times a week for three hours of dialysis. She was not married and had one daughter, twelve years old. Her brother came once in a great while to visit and he would bring her daughter-I think I saw them twice. I met this young lady when the nursing home was under a weather watch, and we were put into a shower room until the weather passed. We were sitting beside each other talking when she said, "I'm scared". I looked at her, and thought *why?* I asked her what she was afraid of and, of course, she said the storm. She asked me if I was scared and when I told her 'No' she asked me why not. I explained that I thought we were all safe, the storm really wasn't that bad; but, the nursing home had to follow rules about weather advisories. In my heart, I knew God was in control no matter what happened. I didn't share my true feelings with her, but, I should have. She held my hand until we were able to return to our rooms. After that we became friends.

It was difficult for anyone to carry on a conversation with this young lady. She would be talking and go to sleep right in the middle of the conversation. I didn't know if it was her medication or the dialysis. I didn't understand, and it was frustrating at times. I checked in on her every day. If she were awake: we would talk, go to therapy together, play bingo or just sit in the hallway. Therapy was trying to get her to use her leg, but, it hurt to the point of bringing her to tears then she would give up. I was asked to accompany her and encourage her to do more and work through the pain. I didn't know what I could say or do, but, I tried.

Over the next couple of months, my companionship with this young lady was beginning to become somewhat of a problem for her, for me, and the nurses. She wouldn't do or go anywhere unless I was with her. For instance, when there was a storm warning, all residents were ushered into the bathrooms away from windows. However, one time she wouldn't go without me. There were two rooms in the shower room: the first room was an entrance room; the second room was where the showers and tubs were. A nurse went to put this young lady into the second room without me and she started fighting with the nurse, and I mean, physically fighting. The nurse looked at me, and I could see she was pretty upset. So upset that if looks could have killed, I'd be dead. I talked the young lady into doing what the nurse was telling her to do and reluctantly she complied. After that, the young lady was upset with me.

The next episode happened when another lady resident and I went to play bingo. We stopped by the youngster's room, but, she was sleeping so we didn't wake her up. When she woke up, she came into bingo and chastised me for not waking her. I wanted to be her friend, but, I wasn't her keeper. It was time for us to talk. She apologized, and then said she wanted to be with me because I had a big support group and she didn't have anybody. I felt bad for her; but, I couldn't fill her emptiness, and her dependency on me bothered me. I suggested she call some of her friends and see if they would visit. I explained I wasn't staying in the nursing home forever and she should not depend on me for her only companionship. That idea wasn't in her best interest. The youngster took my advice and called a friend of hers who did come to visit. When I left, I took her phone number. After I arrived home, I called her. I wondered how she was doing. I prayed she was well.

A black man, slender in stature, about 5'10" tall, said to be a minister, checked into the home in need of therapy due to back surgery. His room was right across the hall from mine. He turned out to be a strange character. At first, he was visited by men and women coming from Church on Sundays. On occasion, he would leave with these people and not come back for a day or two. Then, when he did come back, he would give therapy a hard time. Eventually they discharged him from their schedules. His wife would come to visit, and stay for days. She slept in his bed and he slept in a chair. I couldn't keep up with the shenanigans. It was like "Payton Place". The minister claimed to be homeless, and that was why his wife would stay several nights at a time with him at the nursing home.

A CNA told me the minister was talking to another patient about the Bible and asked if I would be interested in doing a Bible study with him. I declined because I thought his beliefs and mine were not in any way in the same ballpark. I'm not sure if she understood me; but, I'm sure she did later on.

One day the woman we thought to be his wife was in his room, she had been staying there. A nurse came back to tell him someone was waiting for him at the front door. Then she walked over to me and said she didn't know what to do; the woman in his room was, she thought, his wife; and, the woman at the front door said she was his wife. They all left and never came back. He left his computer and everything. Weird or what!!

The young man the black minister was talking to about the Bible had fallen off a roof and broken his hip. He was in Harbor Towne for rehab. A therapist asked me if I would stop by his room and talk to him. I guess she thought I might be able to give him a moral boost; he was terribly depressed and lonely. His family lived down south somewhere. I was uncomfortable with the request, but, I said I would see what I could do.

At the same time, a lady came in on the wing my room is on and south of me by one room. She is a victim of an automobile accident; broken leg, pelvis and hip. She is in a lot of pain and extremely uncomfortable. Once again therapy came to me and asked me to visit with her. I'm not real sure why I'm being asked to make visits to different patients, but, I guess I can do it. I was asked to share my story and show them my injuries; so, during my wandering around the building, I stopped in and introduced myself to the new patient. We talked for a long while. She had been a postal worker until the accident. She shared her accident with me, and I shared mine with her. After our talk that first day, she shared with me later on that she felt as if she had been acting like 'such a baby'. I certainly disagreed with her. Her injuries were just as painful and moving around was just as uncomfortable for her as mine were for me. She ended up staying at Harbor Towne a couple of months and we became pretty close friends. We encouraged each other along with some of the other patients. Both of us tried to encourage the young lady with the broken leg and kidney problems. I couldn't image going through everything she was going through at her young age. The postal victim and I were fairly close in age. Her children were grown, like mine. I believe she ended up being disabled because walking became a real chore for her.

She loved to play bingo though, and after she healed to the point of being able to get around with a walker fairly well; her sister would pick her up and take her to the bingo halls. I got a kick out of her.

If someone brought in food from the outside world or had cooked something in therapy, we shared. The food at Harbor Towne was better than Parkside; but, still not like home. The service left a lot to be desired. Breakfast would be served anywhere from 7:30 a.m. to 9:30 a.m. and dinner was usually not on time either. After the mail lady went home, I missed her for quite a while. I felt everyone around me was going home--except me. I did call her a couple of times. She was having physical therapy come to her home. I lost track of her for a little while; then, probably a year later, she and my favorite therapist from Harbor Towne came to visit me at the Lutheran Home. I loved the visit. I learned she was home doing fairly well at home; while I was in another nursing home following another operation.

After the mail lady was released to go home, the young man who fell off a roof and broke his hip was moved into her room. I was again urged to visit with him, so I went. He was experiencing a rough time. Apparently, his family and girlfriend did come up to stay with him for a while, but they wanted to stay at Harbor Towne with him. They wanted to sleep in the day room, and his girlfriend wanted to sleep in bed with him. How that would have worked for them with his broken hip…I couldn't imagine. The officials at the nursing home discouraged all of them from staying at the home overnight. I woke up one morning and his family had packed him up and took him home. He was in so much pain; that seemed like a bad decision on their part. Oh well, it was his decision and I prayed everything worked out for him.

Among some of my other friends was a rather large lady who came in from having a knee replaced. When she arrived she was so heavy she couldn't get in and out of bed without help. I felt so sorry for her. The knee replacement didn't help; but, I'm sure her weight had a lot to do with the knee going out. She probably stayed two or three months; and within that time she got her weight down quite a bit. She was very proud of her accomplishments. We were all happy for her. And she received encouragement to keep up her good work even after she went home.

There were a couple of other ladies that I have fond memories of; one black lady I thought was super. I don't remember why she was there; but, she retired from an auto factory. I think she either had a knee or hip replaced and was in therapy. She had real short, curly hair, always wore a hat, and sang all the time. She was a jolly old soul. However, she and another black lady, who lived at the other end of the hallway, got into an argument that almost turned into a physical battle. I believe, it was due to a difference of personalities and ideas. That verbal battle upset my friend quite a bit and she went home shortly after that.

Another lady, who lived at the home, was a white lady, exceptionally heavy, could not walk so she rode a scooter all the time; and, wore newsboy hats every day. She told me her granddaughter got her into wearing the hats; they were quite appropriate for her too. We became friends, but, not close. She didn't get close with anyone. She said when she did get close with someone, they would die and, unfortunately, that is just what happened. A lady came in across the hall from the newsboy lady, and they became friends real fast. The lady was acting okay one day and the next thing we knew she passed away. Newsboy took it hard and began distancing herself from me and others.

A lot of people came into Harbor Towne and a lot of people left; they either passed on or went home. Getting used to death on a regular basis was not and never will be an easy thing to do. My faith helped me through. I watched, listened, sometimes visited, and prayed for the failing. I got to a point where I could tell when someone was ready to go live with Jesus and it actually wasn't a sad moment for them.

I did think it strange when a patient would come in for therapy and say, "I don't want to stay in a room where someone has died". I guess I never actually thought of it quite like that; someone has died in every room of a nursing home.

Wayne usually tried to lighten the days up when he was visiting me; nursing homes can be pretty depressing. He teased the CNAs which, of course, they liked. He also teased some of the residents; one lady was giving the CNAs a hard time whining, and trying to get out of her bed without assistance which she could not do without falling; so, they had her lying on her bed in the hallway so the CNAs could keep a better eye on her. Wayne and I passed by her on our way to the door, and out of the blue, Wayne said, "Hi Sweetheart, want to have sex?" The CNAs jaw dropped open, her eyes got real wide, and she gasped. She looked at Wayne, and then at Sweetheart, who was now quiet, and had a grin on her face from ear to ear. Everyone started laughing--even Sweetheart. Wayne distracted her from whining and being restless; plus, he got a laugh out of everyone, which was a good thing. He basically de-stressed the situation with Sweetheart.

The other comical thing that happened was with an elderly lady who was a little over four feet tall, walked with a walker, and was deaf. I don't know if she read lips or what, but, she did not talk just grunted. She would look at you nod, and smile if you smiled at her first. She would not allow anyone clean her room, make her bed, or take care of her laundry. She insisted she would do it. One evening Wayne was pushing me out to the front door because he was leaving after visiting most of the day. Shorty was coming down the hallway toward us with her laundry. She had a hospital gown on with a bed jacket over the top. She turned in front of us to go into the utility room; and, we had to chuckle. Shorty's bed jacket only went to her waist, the hospital gown was open in the back, and she didn't have anything on underneath her gown except her slippers. I heard Wayne chuckle under his breath, "Oh no…" A CNA, who was walking toward us a little way behind Shorty, had a smile on her face and said, "It is what it is…she thinks she is covered." Wayne shook his head, smiled, and said with a chuckle, "I know, it just wasn't a sight I expected to see".

On Halloween, the home was open to the children, grandchildren, and friends of the residents and employees. Before the children came into the home, the residents were ushered into the dining room where we were given candy to hand out to the children as they paraded past us. I wheeled into the dining hall in my wheelchair, found an empty area by a table and parked.

Shortly after I parked, this elderly lady came walking past me giving me real nasty looks and was mumbling to herself. I watched her as she looked at me, and I was wondering what I had done. Then, I heard her say, "That's mine!" It dawned on me then that I was sitting in her place at the dinner table. Apparently, that was a BIG No No…the residents had their places where they sat each and every day, and no one dare take them. I was just about to move, when another lady came by, took her by the hand, and told her it was okay for me to sit where I was, and she could sit somewhere else. The little old lady still looked at me with a disturbed look on her face.

I think more candy was eaten by the residents than was given out to the children, but, it was fun. The CNAs dressed up in costumes too. One of my favorite girls came by and had a picture taken with me. It was a new and different experience for me. I was certainly learning.

My first Thanksgiving, 2006, away from home was at Harbor Towne. A lady friend from church, and the Pastor's wife came to visit often, and when the holidays rolled around they decorated my room for me. I really appreciated their thoughtfulness. There were many other residents who did not have anyone to spend the holidays with. Some of the nurses and CNAs would bring decorations in for those people and they would buy gifts for them as well. Those situations were heart breaking. I was so blessed to have had so many supporters. My lady friends also brought me food, books, and games. They made sure I had everything I needed. Thanksgiving Day the cooks fixed turkeys and all the trimmings. It was very good. If I remember correctly, my mother-in-law, Wayne's aunt, and Wayne were my guests that day; and it definitely was a day for Thanksgiving…I was alive and I had all my parts.

Christmas, 2006, was also spent at Harbor Towne. Again, my lady friends from church decorated my room for the occasion which was truly appreciated. This time we reserved the day room for everyone to bring in food, and some gifts. There were at least twelve of us plus a couple of residents came in and ate with us too. I thought we had an enjoyable Christmas considering my situation and where we were. I was very happy to have everyone come, visit, and share the delicious food; it was comforting. God has been gracious to me and Wayne.

Chapter XII

After the holidays everyone got back into the swing of things, and the home was operating at full staff again. Then the flu hit. There was no escaping it either, and, of course, I got it too. The residents had to eat in their rooms, staff was wearing face masks and gloves, and visitors were cautioned about visiting residents. The CNAs were so busy taking care of sick people I suggested they put my garbage can next to my bed, put a wash tub on top of it, and let me take care of myself until they could return. And, that was what they did. I felt sorry for the girls running around from one room to the next, everyone was so sick. That, too, eventually passed.

In January, 2007, I received a letter from the State of Michigan deeming me disabled and unable to work. I read that letter and said, "Humm…that wasn't my plan, but, I guess its okay." I had in my head that I would return to work someday; however, it had been almost a year though and I was bed and wheelchair bound. Not to mention going through operation after operation. I kept telling people I would return to work; and, Wayne couldn't believe I thought that. My perception of what I was going through was a little off.

When I regained my strength and was virus free, therapy continued. I had two favorite therapists that I dealt with on a daily basis even though all of the therapy team was likeable and pleasant to work with. My occupational therapist worked on my left hand and arm daily--massaging and strengthening. My physical therapist put me through the paces of attempting to walk and put weight on my leg. She looked on the computer for survival statistics of accidents like mine and she whispered to me, "You are a very lucky person." I was thinking *blessed* was a more accurate description. While in therapy, I was having problems with my right tibia. When I put pressure on the leg, it was okay; but, when I took the pressure off my leg, there was sharp shooting pain. I tried to stand three times, but the pain was too intense.

I went back to the doctor for more x-rays; and, what do you know, another operation was scheduled. During this operation they are going to put an external fixator on my right tibia. This one will look different than the one on the left leg. It will be two halos held together with adjustable rods; and, the pins will actually go through my bones. This fixator was uncomfortable and the pins hurt. The rods were adjusted every day to pull the two broken bones together encouraging them to knit and heal. Wayne ended up doing most of the adjusting; because, the nurses didn't want to hurt me. Eventually, a younger, more adventurous nurse did help him. She was one of the nurses who was fascinated with my wounds. She would change the bandages and we would look at them trying to figure out which was bone, and muscle, and tendons, and tissues. I have to admit, I was fascinated too.

While I was staying at Harbor Towne, I had gone for a couple bone graphs--where the bone was scrapped from my hip bones, mixed with I don't know what, and applied to the breaks. In the past, doctors had used cadaver bone, and synthetic bone; but, neither of those procedures worked. Plus, while in the operating room, the doctors were suppose to exchange the rod that was in my left femur. The rod in my leg had been inserted June, 2006, and apparently, was too small. The doctors wanted a larger, permanent rod connected with two pins in my left knee. Then, they were to manipulate my leg to ensure it was as straight as it could be--for the time being. Needless to say, recovery was painful.

Every time I left Harbor Towne to go to a doctor appointment, I was extended good luck wishes by everyone as they saw me leave. It gave me a warm feeling to know people, who barely knew me, were wishing me well. When I returned to the home, I received the same friendly greetings.

Probably six weeks later I had another operation. During each operation, the muscle flap on my left leg would be opened, cleaned out, and stitched back up. There were three plates and pins just above the ankle, plus, the external fixator. Work on my right tibia included tying the muscles, tendons, and tissues together with, what I called, metal twisty ties. The wound was left open to heal from the inside out using a wet-to-dry bandaging method. The doctor said I could put full weight on my leg. I was excited! Full weight meant I could return to therapy; and, using a walker, I could gently hop a little way up and down the hallway. It certainly would be hard work, but it also was considered progress.

While in the hospital, the afternoon nurse was unable to change my bandages before her shift ended. However, she told the nurse coming on duty that she would stay and do it. He told her he would take care of my bandages and she didn't have to stay. As they came down the hall, I could hear them talking back and forth about who was going to change my bandages. They both came in the room, and the first nurse started changing my left leg. The second nurse stood, watching for a minute, and then asked if he could change the other leg. There was a nurse working on each leg. I got a kick out of those two nurses. My injuries were fascinating to those people. They would get excited to see them. I have to admit, by watching, I was learning a lot. I don't remember staying in the hospital very long, maybe a couple of days before I went back to Harbor Towne.

I was excited to be able to put full weight on my leg; however, my excitement didn't last. The same day I returned to the nursing home, Wayne and I were visiting, and I asked him to assist me in going to the bathroom. Reluctantly, he agreed. We were in the bathroom; he lifted and turned me into position, and I got the right leg external fixator caught under the lip of the toilet. I pulled my leg out, put *full weight* on it, when I felt the twisty ties pop! Pop! Pop! Pop! I screamed in pain! Wayne fearfully asked, "What did you do?" All I could say was, "My leg! My leg! Wayne put me back in the wheelchair, saw all the blood soaking my sock, and ran out of the room for the nurse! I wheeled myself back into my room, and looked at my leg. When I saw the bandages and my sock, my heart sunk. With Wayne's help, the CNAs and nurse put me in bed, the fire department was called and an ambulance. The nurse took off the bandages to check the wound and to determine whether the bones had moved or not. She didn't think so, but I was rushed to the hospital for a doctor to look at the wound. Since it was late, Wayne drove himself to the hospital and met me in the emergency room. After x-rays doctor determined I *only* popped some of the wires they had *just* put in. He took out two wires, tightened two wires, bandaged me back up, and sent me home. It apparently, wasn't a big deal to them. It sure felt like a big deal to me--mega pain! This had been the story of my life these days; two steps forward and one step back or three steps forward and two steps back. Oh well, at least the bones were still in place--that was a good thing. Praise God!

I was bed ridden for a few more days, and pretty sore from the previous nights' activity; no better time to read the book Wayne bought me, '90 Minutes In Heaven' by Don Piper. I was surprised at how close my situation sounded to Mr. Pipers. I didn't see heaven though, and I was disappointed. I didn't see the angels either; but, I know they were with me. I was also surprised at how many surgeries he had endured. I called my insurance case worker and was telling her about the book; and, that Mr. Piper had something like thirty-five operations. She hesitated a minute and said, "You've had thirty-two". I didn't believe her, just seemed unreal to me. She assured me by saying she had just finished counting all the operations and there were thirty-two. Like I said earlier, realizing all I had been through hadn't sunk into my brain. And, it was early in the healing process.

Sitting in bed one evening I felt the hematoma that had developed from the accident. It was located under my left arm, running horizontally, and the size of a large hot dog. I was told it would eventually be absorbed into my body and not to worry about it. That was easy for someone else to say. Anyway, while checking it out, I found a small lump in my left breast. *Oh great, something else to deal with!* I called the nurse she checked me, and said she would make an appointment for me to have an ultrasound. With that, she left. A few minutes later se returned and said instead of an ultrasound they would do a blood test in the morning. I was more comfortable with that decision. The blood work was ordered stat so I didn't have to wait long for the results; which were, *Thank the Lord*, negative for cancer. Those results were a welcomed relief! The blood clot was breaking up and moving to different areas. I didn't think I could handle any more health problems. I was already wondering just how much more my heart would take. I tried to keep in mind that the Lord doesn't give anyone any more than they can handle. However, I thought, I might have been given an oversized plate.

The problems continued to come. God, apparently, wasn't finished with me. I developed a small bulge on the right side of my stomach, just to the right of the belly button. I summoned the nurse to look at it. She determined it was a hernia. My thoughts went back to the plastic surgeon, and her comment about fixing a hernia when she removed the muscle from my abdomen. The next day the bulge was bigger, and I called the hospital for a referral to a doctor to examine it. Following the examination, I had a surgery date to repair the hernia. An EMTS person, inadvertently, told me that it was going to be a painful operation. I didn't know; but, I thought all of my operations were pretty painful. Anyway, the operation took place; the doctor put a screen in my stomach to cover the herniated area, and the area where the muscle had been removed. Then, he glued the wound back together. Something different, I had never had glue before. By the way, the EMTS person was right--painful. I was given a pillow to hold in front of me and grasp when I coughed. Of course, I coughed.

One evening, while sitting alone by the nurse's station; it was all quiet, and the nurse on duty was getting her med cart ready to pass meds. She was a plump young lady, short in stature, and dark brown hair—pleasant. I didn't see her often as she worked contingent; so, when, out of the blue, she said, "Sandy, would you pray for me?" I was puzzled. I looked at her and asked, "Why, is there something going on?" She answered, "No, I just know you pray and I'd like for you to pray for me". I didn't know her name, which I asked for, and told her I'd be more than happy to put her in my prayers. I was surprised and honored that she asked me to pray for her. I thought her request was quite extraordinary—especially of me.

Things, quite often, didn't go easily; there were lots of bumps in the road. Harbor Towne had one CNA who had quite an attitude. And, we had a problem on her last day of work. I was certainly glad it was her last day too. I had been confined to a bed for so long that when my assigned CNA got me out of bed and into a wheelchair, that was where I wanted to stay. This was what I had been doing for a while. However, this particular day, my assigned CNA got me up and about midmorning; she returned a short time later stating she was leaving for a while. If I wanted to get back into bed, she would help me before she left. I asked how long she was going to be gone, but she didn't know. I told her I wanted to stay in the wheelchair. I was certain if I needed to get back into bed, someone would help me. I hadn't had any problems getting help in the past.

I didn't anticipate this one CNA having the attitude *ain't my job.* Four o'clock in the evening rolled around and my CNA had not returned. I had to go to the bathroom; and, I asked a young lady to help me get back into bed so I could use the bed pan. She agreed, to help put me in bed; however, she needed help. She asked the CNA with attitude to help her. Attitude's comment was, "No, she refused earlier to go back to bed, she can just wait for her CNA now". I was shocked at her comment. I didn't think I had *refused* to go back to bed; I had been given an option. Anyway, I went back to my room; and, the nurse came in said they were short handed, and she needed everyone on the floor to cooperate. I understood, but, I had been in my wheelchair all day and I had to go to the bathroom. They finally agreed to take me to the bathroom. It took three ladies to lift me to the toilet and put me back in the wheelchair. By doing it that way, it took more woman power and time than just putting me in bed and giving me the bed pan.

A couple hours later my CNA came back. I was upset with her for telling people I *refused* to get back in bed before she left. I informed her that if I could do things for myself, I would not be asking anyone for help. It was humiliating having strangers help with my every need; and I did not appreciate a caretaker who gave me a hard time when I needed help. Of course, she said she didn't tell anyone I *refused* to go back to bed that morning. Consequently, that conversation went nowhere. That was the first time I had felt angry for being helpless and having to beg someone to assist me. I thought my CNA saw my frustration. She apologized, and put me in bed for the night. I didn't know if the CNA with attitude admitted to what happened; but, it was her last night at Harbor Towne so it didn't matter. I was glad to see her leave, and I did wonder if she was going to go back to work at a nursing home in her new location.

Chapter XIII

Following the above incident with Attitude, it seemed my physical therapy was stepped up a bit. I was shown how to use a slide board to get from the bed to the wheelchair or onto my own potty chair and back into bed. That gave me a little more independence. My therapy seemed to be moving along fairly well considering. On Saturdays the therapy people were different, the regulars worked Monday through Friday, and the weekends were part timers. On Saturdays an older man would come in and work with me. He asked continually if I was writing my book. I would just say "No, maybe some day." He asked if I had kept notes or a journal on everything I had went through, and he encouraged me to start writing a journal from where I was at in my recovery at that time. I couldn't believe people thought I should write a book. How was I any different from other accidents? I didn't quite understand why everyone thought I had a story to tell. Being called a "Miracle" was also difficult to swallow. I felt that I had to live up to a much higher standard and expectation of other people.

Pastor came to visit me one day in March, and during our visit, I said I would be coming home on Mother's Day, 2007. I didn't think I would be in perfect condition; but, I was positively determined to get home--even for an afternoon. I was becoming pretty independent with everything therapy had me doing daily; like, board transfers and using a walker. Even with two external fixators, I was getting around fairly well. For the most part, though, I was confined to a wheelchair; and, I still had a couple of months before May, which would mark a year since the initial accident. I hadn't been home at all over this time period; so, I was extremely hopeful. I knew they wouldn't be sending me home until the fixators were removed and everything looked acceptable. The removal of the halo fixator from my right leg was the next operation. It felt as if it had been on my leg for an eternity! I was so glad to be getting rid of that fixator, and I prayed the leg was healed.

After the usual round of x-rays, Wayne and I were waiting in the examining room for doctors to look at the pictures, when an extremely excited intern actually jumped through the door and exclaimed, "It's healed! Your leg is healed!" I was as relieved as the intern was excited. He continued to say, "Now, let's get the other leg healed!" Unfortunately, the left leg wasn't doing as well; but, I took what I could get. The intern looked at my left leg; and, with a serious tone in his voice, said, "This will take a long time". My idea of a long time and his, however, were two different ideas. I was sent back to the nursing home for more rehab. Patience wasn't one of my better qualities, but, I had to learn; *in God's time not mine.*

In April, 2007 the fixator on my left leg was removed. Again, I was told to *walk on it,* and with the assistance of a walker, I did. I didn't put all of my weight on my legs even though I was told I could. I used my arms to hold me; because using my left leg was painful. The week of Mother's Day, 2007 arrived; and, I wanted to go to church that Sunday. My daughter and daughter-in-law arranged, without Wayne knowing, to pick me up and take me to church. I was so excited. Therapy took me outside a few times to practice getting in and out of a car. We used the therapist's car. My mother-in-law didn't think it was a good idea for me to leave the home. She was afraid I would get injured or an infection might find its way into my wounds; but, therapy said I could go and that was what I was going to do. There were going to be concerns. I had to be cognizance of every move I made.

Sunday came, and the kids were there to pick me up, and away we went. When we arrived at church, I had to enter via an outside elevator; which was very old and rickety. The ushers helped and I made it. A friend of ours went upstairs to get Wayne, who did not know I was coming. When he saw me, he started to cry along with a couple of ushers. Church was full. We sat in the back because of the wheelchair. Wayne asked if I wanted to take communion, which, I did. He said we would go up last to avoid any confusion. We wheeled up to the Pastor who, before he gave me the bread, said, "I'm not supposed to say this at this time, but, you said you would be home on Mother's Day and even though it's not to stay, you are here." After I had received communion, Wayne turned me around to return to our pew and the congregation began applauding. *I was taken back!* I didn't know what to do or how to react. The Pastor took a minute after we had returned to our seats to explain to the rest of the congregation that it was my first time home and to church in a year due to the accident. I was so moved by everyone's reactions to my being in church. It was so special to Wayne and me and meant so very much.

Following church, Wayne said we needed to wait until the crowd thinned out before we left. I was sitting next to the door where Pastor stood to shake hands and wish everyone God's Blessings and a good week. There were many people stopping by me crying, shaking my hand, giving me hugs, and telling me what a *Miracle* I was. One man came past crying and said, "I just want to touch you". He touched my shoulder with his finger and walked on wiping the tears from his eyes. It was all unbelievable. We never expected a reception such as that.

Lord, was all this the answer to a prayer I said in January of 2006? Were you working to answer my own prayer through me? I certainly was not sure how to handle all of these emotional people. I told a few people at the nursing home what happened in church that day; and they got emotional right along with me. I understood it wasn't me so much as the miracle God had worked using me and my family.

It was either June or July 2007, when I did get to go home. What a great day that was! Two of the therapists came to my house to do a home study; making sure my home was safe for me to return to. One of the therapists entered my kitchen and said, "Looks like something out of Better Homes and Gardens." That was a great compliment! They made a long list of items I would need in order for me to come home. I was approved to use a walker inside the house and a wheelchair for outside and distances. The wheel chair wouldn't go through my bathroom door anyway nor could I get upstairs.

Prior to my leaving Harbor Towne, the staff gave me going home/good luck gifts. I received three different bags of truffles; which were absolutely delicious, and some nice lotions. The best gift of all was—a bed pan decorated with flowers and signed by everyone. I was so touched--it was great! I went looking for my angel of a nurse who had a hard time saying good-bye to her special patients. She hid in the office, waiting for me to leave; but, I found her. We both cried, hugged, and I left. It was a happy/sad ending at Harbor Towne.

Wayne had a hospital bed put in our dining room for me to sleep on because I could not negotiate the stairs. I used the full bathroom we had downstairs. I took showers in the tub with the help of a shower chair. A friend from church set up a schedule of volunteers who brought in meals a couple of times a week. I didn't have to cook and Wayne didn't have to cook for me. The church was wonderful; everyone was awesome! Some of the ladies would stay and talk with me; which, I loved! Coming home, after being gone for ten months it was, how should I say it, strange? Wayne had his own way of doing things which was much different from mine. The pots and pans were in different cupboards. My towels were in different cupboards…in different rooms. Example, my kitchen towels were in the bathroom. He did laundry differently too. He vacuumed and wet mopped my floors every day. I had a cat, and Wayne didn't like all the hair floating around. Plus, I had an open wound where the muscle flap refused to heal closed. I didn't complain; believe me, Wayne kept a pretty clean house.

Wayne and my cat were a story all their own. Tigger was a male, grey tabby about six years old and fifteen pounds. Wayne teased him a lot so my cat didn't like Wayne. After my accident, however, it was just Wayne and Tigger at the house. Tigger stopped sitting in the chair he and I used to sit in all the time. It was *our* chair. And he continued to ignore Wayne.

After a while, Tigger started rolling around on Wayne's feet and would whine. Wayne would pet him; but, he wouldn't get in the chair with him. Then one day, when Wayne came to visit me at the home, he said Tigger had jumped in the chair and laid down next to him. Tigger finally figured if I wasn't coming back, Wayne would have to do. When I did finally return home, Tigger went back to his normal routine--ignoring Wayne completely. He wouldn't even go near him. We had to laugh--Tigger was my cat.

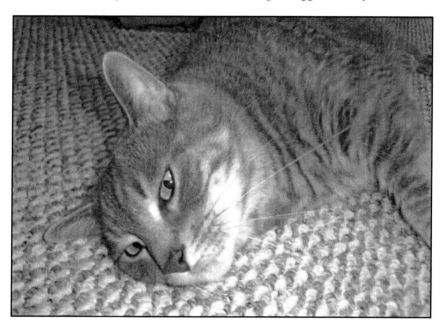

Being home was wonderful; but, was it wasn't what I expected? I was not the same person: I wasn't near as mobile, physically strong, nor did I have near the energy as before the accident. What a rude awakening for me! It was awful! I didn't like being different. I had to learn to do things all over again. I had been waited on hand and foot for almost a year and getting back into the swing of things was a battle. I got up one morning, started the coffee the way I normally did, turned it on; and, realized that I forgot to put the water in the coffee maker. Luckily, I didn't burn it up. I attempted to bake cookies too. We ate them; but, I don't know how or why. They were awful. I wanted to cook; but, I had to give every step some thought on how to do it. My left arm wouldn't turn over, because I could not move it at the elbow. The elbow was fixed in place; which made my arm four inches shorter than my right. Since I used to be totally left handed, except for writing, doing things in the kitchen was quite an adjustment. I had to make conscious efforts to use my left hand/arm and not favorite it.

I couldn't vacuum, mop floors, dust, or shake rugs. I hadn't figured out how to hold a mop; and, I would lose my balance when I tried to use the vacuum cleaner. Making the bed was an awful challenge. I hopped around the bed like a monkey jumping around on the ground. I couldn't put full weight on my leg without pain. I had a terrible time lifting the mattress to tuck in the sheets--my strength wasn't there. To stand at the sink and wash my face and brush my teeth was painful. Any weight on my leg sent sharp shooting pain up my leg. Frustrating, very frustrating! But, I didn't complain. I never said anything to Wayne--he worried about me enough, and I didn't want to add to his worry.

I didn't have clothes downstairs and I was a little tired of wearing Wayne's shorts and tees. I wanted warmer clothes, and, clothes to wear to church. I would give Wayne a description of what I wanted out of my closet and he went upstairs to retrieve it for me. *Oh, my gosh! He just doesn't get it! I have to get upstairs and retrieve some clothes that I can wear!* One afternoon I waited until Wayne left for a while, then I crawled upstairs on my butt, pulling my walker with me. I picked out the clothes I wanted and crawled, on my butt, back down the steps. After sneaking up and down the stairs, I hoped I had gotten enough exercise that day to get a good night's sleep without leg spasms.

One afternoon, my lady friends from church stopped by the house to visit; and, they retrieved a variety of clothes from my closet for me. Praise God. Coming home brought a new set of challenges and frustrations. It took over an hour the first time I put my pierced earrings in. I couldn't get a necklace on without using magnets to hook the chains or Wayne hooked it for me. Lord, how I prayed for tolerance and patience.

Three times a week a therapist came to the house. His mission was to strengthen my core muscles and legs. We were talking one afternoon, and he told me about one of his other clients that had problems similar to mine with her foot and ankle. She, like me, could not move the ankle up and down and could not wear heels any more or even get on high top boots. He told me how upset she was about it; and, I told him to share my story with her. When I got home I gave away three garbage bags full of almost brand new shoes that I could no longer wear. I knew how bad I felt having to get rid of most all my shoes, and not knowing what I was going to be able to wear or not wear. I hoped my therapist told his young client she wasn't alone. I really could sympathize with her.

After doing therapy at home for a month or two, my leg began bowing out as if I was bow-legged. I went back to the doctor, and, yup, another operation was scheduled. All my walking to encourage the bones to heal did just the opposite. I cracked the bones above and below the plates. I was in a lot of pain so I kept taking pain meds to walk. The meds took the sharp bite out of the pain which made it tolerable for me; and, masked the reason for the pain. I didn't realize the extent of the damage.

I went into the hospital thinking I would come out with a boot or a cast and the plates would be out. Well, that didn't happen. I came out of surgery without two of the plates still in my leg, and another external fixator. Needless to say, I was pretty disappointed. I stayed one night in the hospital and was sent home. While at the hospital, I had walked up and down the hallway with my walker and went into the bathroom by myself. It was presumed that I was doing well; so, I was released to go home. By the time Wayne and I arrived home, I was in so much pain it was unreal. The pain pill I had taken did absolutely nothing. I sat rocking back and forth trying to control myself while Wayne talked to the insurance case worker and intake at the Lutheran Home. If Wayne couldn't get me into the Lutheran Home, I would have to go back to the hospital. Our insurance case worker finally agreed to let me go into the nursing home, if a room was available.

The Lutheran Home was located right down the road from where we lived, and the girls were waiting by the door when we pulled up. The intake lady came out to me first, and I immediately started crying. I was in so much *pain*. Several girls helped me into a wheelchair and down a hallway to wait for maintenance and housekeeping to ready my room. Once in the room, I was put to bed and the head nurse came in to go over the rules and to mark, on a sketch of a body, all my scars, marks, and tattoos. The only thing I had was scars and she said, "I'm running out of room to put these," and I responded, "me too". The pain was so great and the meds were not working--I couldn't have been more miserable.

The CNAs took me out of bed and put me in a recliner hoping I could get more comfortable. I kept telling Wayne the doctor had to have broken my bones and reset them. Wayne kept denying the allegations. I was in so much pain--I didn't believe him. Around 10:00 p.m. I told Wayne to go home. His fussing with me only upset him and me. Aprell was there for a while too--until I told her to go home. The CNAs were changing shifts so they put me back in bed, and put ice on my leg. The cold just about sent me through the roof, and lying down didn't help either. I asked to be put back in the chair and covered up. I was alone. I relaxed enough to go to sleep. If the pain hadn't subsided, the nursing home was about to send me to the hospital. Thankfully, I fell asleep and I didn't wake up until about 10:00 a.m. the next day.

The Chaplain came to visit with me early that afternoon. He was a motorcycle rider himself and had been in a nasty accident some twenty years earlier. He shared his story with me, and, I shared my story with him. I was relieved to learn the Chaplain was still a motorcycle rider. I thought, *there's still hope for me.*

Later in the afternoon, my neighbor came over and introduced herself to me and brought me a wrapped bar of soap. Jane was in her ninety's, wheelchair bound, and very hard of hearing. However, she heard everything I went through during the night, and she felt sorry for me. She brought me a bar of soap as a consolation gift. She was cute. Before we became too acquainted, I was moved to another room--the next day. The room I was in had been promised to another lady before my arrival, so I had to move. Well, soon as Jane realized I was gone she had a fit. She came to my new room and said, "They moved you! Why did they move you? They had no right to do that! I like you and you need to tell them to move you back!" then she left. Stunned, Wayne and I looked at each other and chuckled. I had only seen Jane once, and that was when she brought me the soap. How funny was that? Later on, I would see her in the hallway and she would smile, and say, "Hello, crip" (short for cripple). I got a kick out of Jane. She was known for her 'tatting'. The nursing home displayed a picture of her needle work in the hallway. Jane was also a self-appointed caretaker of the birds the Lutheran Home had in one of their dayrooms; and, pop can tab collector.

Every nursing home must have a 'Grandma'. The Lutheran Home had a 'Grandma' too. I met her while I was sitting in a day room looking at a magazine. I was in my wheelchair with my left leg up and extended. Someone went past me in a wheelchair, stopped, and said hello. Grandma was coming from around the passerby; she spied my foot and made a bee line over to me. She looked at my foot intently. Then, without any warning, she grabbed my big toe and shook it! I yelled "No, don't touch!" Grandma looked up at me, and let loose of my toe. She backed up a little, looked at me again, looked back at my toe, and reached for it again! A CNA, who came out of nowhere, grabbed Grandma's wheelchair and whooshed her off apologizing as they left. I chuckled. She didn't hurt me either time; she caught me off guard. She was curious and probably hadn't seen anything like that before. Another lesson learned. I believe Grandma was 100 years old. She tooled around the home in her own little world, ignored everyone and everything around her. I was told she was the mother of twelve children. If she could tell you all she had seen throughout her years, it would have been quite the history lesson. Amazing! These two ladies, Jane and Grandma, were my first acquaintances at the Lutheran Home, and I was already enjoying their presence.

The Lutheran Home was the Cadillac of nursing homes. Every resident had their own room. You did share a bathroom, but, you did have your own medicine cabinet to put personal items in. Some of the rooms had pretty wall paper on at least one wall. All the rooms are carpeted including the hallways. Carpeting made for quieter surroundings. It didn't stop the residents from yelling; but, it was a much homier feel. In the summer, you could get an air conditioner put in your window; otherwise, the air was at the nurses' stations and the porches. There was a beautiful little chapel with forty-seven 'church mice' carved in the woodwork all around the room. Beautiful stained glass windows were actually brought here from Germany. The organ was massive and also just beautiful. Church services were held on Fridays. Everyone could get the services on their room TV's if they didn't want or couldn't attend in the chapel.

In all the day rooms, there was old and new furniture; pictures and glassware from past residents. It reminded me of what a grandmother's home looked like maybe forty years ago. The birds, that Jane took care of, were in one of the day rooms. Residents were sat by their cages so they could watch them flit about. One big glass and screened in cage had doves and finches. An outside company came in to take care of these birds every three months.

Then there were two other cages. One had a parrot and the other had a cockatiel. The parrot could talk, "here kitty, kitty, kitty" and some other things that have escaped my memory. The cockatiel would whistle at girls, give you kisses, and let you take her for walks around the home, while sitting on your shoulder. Jane didn't want anyone doing anything with those birds. If you did something she disapproved of, you would certainly hear about it in no uncertain terms. Her one main pet peeve was people who gave the birds scrambled eggs. "Don't give the birds scrambled eggs! "It makes them poop green!"

Eunice Hansen, a resident since about the late 1980's also took care of the birds-- usually when Jane was not around. Eunice was the lady who would give the birds 'scrambled eggs'. Eunice didn't care what Jane said. She said eggs wouldn't hurt the birds at all.

My second room at the Lutheran home was at the very north end of 'A' wing, and Eunice was second room from the nurses' station, south of me at the other end of the hall. Eunice and I; and, I can't forget Dolly, became good friends. Dolly was a fat little Shih Tzu that Eunice had volunteered to be caretaker of at least eleven years earlier. They were inseparable roommates. Dolly would patrol 'A' wing, unless Eunice was somewhere else in the building…Dolly was never far away. Unless, of course, Dolly didn't want to be where Eunice was; then she would go home and wait for Eunice to return. Wayne picked up some doggy treats for Dolly so we had something to give her when she visited my room. Consequently, we too became pretty good friends.

My first stay at the Lutheran Home lasted for seven months. I got to know a lot of the residents and their families during this time. It was actually a quite comfortable stay. Everyone who worked there was great. The home's resident doctor would come to visit the patients once a month; and, he would arrive at 7:30 a.m. He was young, probably fresh out of school, cocky, and didn't have time to listen to anyone. He would be in and out before you could turn over in bed. My first meeting with him didn't set a very good tone either. I was sleeping when he and the nurse came in, flipped the light on and the nurse announced his arrival. He stood at the bedside for less than a minute. He didn't wait for me to take the bandages off my leg so he could examine it. He just asked a few questions; one being, 'Think you'll ever get on a bike again?' Since I didn't care for his flippant attitude I responded with, "Oh… I might!" He shook his head and left. I thought, *who does he think he is?* He might be a smart person; but, not a patient person to be visiting all these elderly people.

My next visit with this doctor went a little different. In between his visits I had been to my ortho doctor and retrieved several copies of my x-rays; and, I had Wayne bring in my folder of the first x-rays taken which I hung on my bulletin board. This young doctor came in, still in a hurry, and again he didn't wait for me to get up before he went to another patient. I flew out of bed, took the bandages off my leg, and told the CNA "Go get him, please". I was determined that he actually *see* my leg and look at the x-rays. To my surprise, he did come back. He looked at my leg, and was actually fascinated with the fixator. I told him he could look at the x-ray copies on the bulletin board if he liked. After all his oohs and aahs he said, "You really have been through a lot. This is amazing." I responded with, "Yes, I have, thank you." Never saw the young man again. A different physician's assistant came to the home the next month. He was an older, more mature and patient man. We talked a lot about the accident and the procedures being done on my leg.

When I was at Harbor Towne, the doctors had ordered two electric bone stimulators for me to strap onto both my legs. Bone Stimulators are used to encourage the bones to mend via electrical currents. I had gone to the hospital for an operation and when I came back, only one stimulator would work. I used it on my left leg and put the other one away. I couldn't feel the electrical currents; but, I did become a little concerned when a thunder and lightning storm rolled through. I took the stimulator off quickly and waited for the storm to pass through. I didn't want to become a lightning rod.

While at the Lutheran Home, I wore the stimulator a couple of times. I woke up one morning and on the top of my leg, right in the middle, under the fixator bars there was a blister. I asked the physicians assistant about the possibility of the stimulator having caused the blister. He had to do some investigating, but, thought it could have been responsible for the blister. My skin in that area was sensitive and numb so I couldn't feel if it got too hot. That did it for me…no more stimulator…it wasn't doing what it was designed to do anyway. I'm sure Dr. Ebraheim wasn't happy that I wouldn't wear the stimulator; but, it was strapped over the fixator and wasn't touching my leg...I believed that was the reason the stimulator wasn't doing the job it was thought it should do. In most cases, they do help bones heal.

At the home, my days were pretty ordinary--not boring, just routine. Most of the residents woke up in the mornings at around 6:00 a.m.; and, some before that time, but, they normally went to bed before 7:30 p.m. Breakfast was served in the dining room at 7:00 a.m. I always ate in my room. I didn't want to take up space in the dining room because I was a temporary resident; and, the dining room was pretty full to begin with. Besides, I got to sleep in until my food was brought to me at 7:30 a.m. then I could take my time and eat in bed. After breakfast, I would wash up, brush my teeth, do my hair, and head down to the dining room for the 10:00 a.m. activity and coffee time; unless, therapy came after me first. I liked therapy in the mornings or early afternoons because that was when I had the most energy. After about 3:00 p.m., I would tire out. If I didn't sleep the night before, I was worn out all day. Due to leg spasms, I would be up most nights talking to nurses at 2:00 a.m. I would get so tired my eyes looked like 'two burnt holes in a blanket' as my Dad would've said. The leg spasms were due to the scarring and damage to nerves. I struggle with spasms even today.

Therapy at the Lutheran Home was done a little different.ly than at Harbor Towne. I had to start out with occupational as well as physical therapy. I really didn't need occupational therapy, except maybe to use a squishy ball to strengthen my grip. As far as the range of movement in my ring finger and little finger, they were as good as they were going to get. I couldn't make a tight fist with my left hand because those two fingers wouldn't close all the way. I had to be careful when hanging onto items so I didn't drop them. I maxed out in my physical therapy within a few months; but, they let me continue to exercise on my own. The therapists used me as an example to the other residents attempting to encourage them to exercise. I felt self conscious about being an example because I was at least twenty plus years younger than most of the residents. They probably tired just watching me. I ended up doing a lot of talking and becoming friends with most of them.

The nursing home had two computers in a small sitting room off one of the hallways for use by visitors, CNAs, or patients. I used them every day to regain my typing skills. I took an online typing test and discovered my speed was close to the same as it was before the accident; and, typing was a good exercise for my fingers. If I typed for too long, though, my arm would cramp up. I was just relieved I could still type. To pass the time, I spent a lot of time on the computer.

I started playing bingo in the dinning room with the ladies. It was something to do and I helped some of the residents find the numbers and keep up with the caller. At first, I sat with a couple of ladies I became very fond of. One of the ladies gave me a birthday card that read: *This is more than just a card to say Happy Birthday! It's also a handy fan in the event of a hot flash.* It was perfect! I almost wore the card out using it as a fan. After bingo there would be a snack and coffee. Eunice didn't play bingo, but, she came down afterward for the snack and coffee. There were five or six of us who would sit and pass the time in conversation and laughter. Eunice always sat with a friend of hers who didn't do much except watch TV all day every day; and, put bread crumbs outside her window for the squirrels, ducks, geese, and other critters. This friend would come to the dining room for meals and at snack and coffee time to visit with Eunice and Dolly. At first, this lady was okay with me sitting at their table. After a while, she began getting rather testy with me. And, when Wayne would join us, she got even testier. I didn't want to come between the two friends; so, I backed off and went back to the computers instead of sticking around after bingo and visiting.

Another resident told me Eunice's friend acted the same way with her too; but, she figured they were two peas in a pod and didn't want anyone else to interfere in their friendship. I felt bad for this lady because she needed someone to be friends with. And, Eunice lived almost right across the hall from her. I had a conversation with Eunice about her lady friend and how they were being perceived by other residents. I told Eunice I wanted to be friends with her; but, at the same time I didn't want to intrude on their relationship. I ruffled Eunice's feathers a bit and she told me she was friends with whoever wanted to be friends with her. She didn't want anyone thinking she was a one-at-a-time friend type of a person. After our conversation, I was more comfortable hanging around Eunice even though her lady friend felt I was intruding. It was just that lady's way; so, I let her rude comments roll off my back.

Over time, I learned there were some pretty interesting ladies living in the nursing home. Right next door to Eunice was a mentally challenged lady. She had the mentality of maybe a ten year old, but she was actually close to seventy years old when I met her. She was short, and stocky in stature. She could talk when she wanted to. She could scream too. Sometimes the other ladies would get upset with her and be mean to her. She could be very annoying; and, she did have a mean streak in her. I wasn't so sure she knew what she was doing that irritated people though. This lady had an older brother who would visit her every day; sometimes for a minute and at other times for a long while. Eunice said the brother would reminisce with his sister about times when they were youngsters at home. They had a special bond. It was very heartwarming to witness.

On the other side of Eunice was a lady who was always smiling or singing. Her favorite song was "You Are My Sunshine". She didn't like Eunice's other neighbor at all--she didn't want her around. On a Sunday evening, I went to the dining room watch an oldie but goody movie with some of the residents. I sat behind the Sunshine lady and next to the mentally challenged lady. I was talking to Miss Challenge attempting to keep her attention on the movie. However, she started repeatedly hitting her hand on her wheelchair arm. Ms. Sunshine yelled at her to "stop it!" I tried to calm Ms. Sunshine down and encourage Miss Challenge not to slap the arm of her wheelchair. Needless to say, I was not trained in confrontational therapy. Ms. Sunshine turned, attempted to slap Miss Challenge with her open hand. This time it was me that yelled "stop it!." The commotion brought a CNA to rescue Miss Challenge and escorted her back to her room.

The next incident with Ms. Sunshine happened with my husband. He was standing in the day room talking with another man--not paying any attention to anything around him--when Ms. Sunshine came up behind the two men in her wheelchair. She stopped and quietly waited for a few minutes then cleared her throat and said, "Excuse me". Wayne, being the smarty that he could be, turned around and said, "What for? What did you do?" Ms. Sunshine wasn't so sunny and did not like being teased; she retorted back, "NOTHING! I want to get through you *Jackass*!" We all burst out laughing and Wayne came back with, "That's MR. Jackass to you!" It was so unexpected coming from the 'Sunshine Girl'. By the time she got to the hall she lived on, she didn't remember saying anything and even denied it--too comical.

Evelyn was one hundred years old when I arrived at the home. She had lived there as long as Eunice. In her younger day she helped Eunice and Thelma with several craft projects. Now, all she wanted was to go home to the Lord. However, she still had spunk. One evening she was giving the nurse and CNA a hard time so I asked her if she wanted to go to the dining room for the evening activity. She agreed and the nurse thanked me. We were sitting at a table with the other ladies and Evelyn asked for some coffee. The activity leader told her she didn't think there was any coffee made. Evelyn started to get upset. The activity leader said, "Don't get upset, Evelyn, I'll go to the kitchen and see if I can get you some coffee." The activity lady left, Evelyn turned to me and said, "Sometimes you gotta do that to get what you want." I thought to myself, *You little stinker*. Evelyn was old, but, she knew how to work the system. I believe she died at age 103.

One of Eunice's best friends lived in the same hall as we did. Thelma was in her nineties, a very pleasant and friendly lady. She walked around the halls hanging onto the back of her wheelchair pushing it. I was amazed she hardly had any grey in her hair; it was dark, very thick and curly. Thelma, Eunice, and Evelyn in their earlier years made Raggedy Ann and Andy dolls together to sell plus they did other craft projects together. Eunice and Thelma still had a couple of the dolls stored away in their closets. The dolls were made so perfectly and cute.

Thelma would play bingo at a separate table with another lady. This woman was a double amputee; plus, her fingers were very crippled due to arthritis. She would complain that her 'big toe' kept her awake at night. She said it would hurt so bad she couldn't sleep…phantom pain. She was a farmer's wife and the mother of eight adult children…all of whom visited quite often. The ladies used to tell a story of this sweet lady visiting Eunice and Thelma at the Lutheran Home one day during the winter. The snow had begun to fall so she decided she should go home before it got too deep. Well, she got out in the country, in the general direction of her home, and got lost. The snow had changed the look of the countryside and she became confused. She told us, "I made it home, but, I don't know how. Nothing looked familiar to me once the snow covered the ground." Apparently, she did not have a good sense of direction and they always worried about her getting home when she left the Lutheran Home.

Thelma was the mother of one daughter who didn't visit very often. I felt sad for her because she was so proud of her daughter and it appeared to me that the daughter was too busy to give her mother the time her mom would have liked. After bingo was over Thelma and her friend would sometimes join us at our table for a snack and coffee. When all the ladies got together and started talking, it was a wonderful history lesson. It really was amazing to hear about what they had witnessed throughout their lives.

Their stories weren't always about when they were younger, even though those stories were the greatest, they sometimes would come up with cute stories that happened at the home. I was sitting with Eunice and Thelma drinking our coffee one mid-morning when Thelma said, "Last night a young man, one of the student CNAs, asked if he could give me a bath. I thought for a minute…what the heck—and said, 'okay, why not'." She chuckled and said, "He only washed my back." Eunice exclaimed, "Oh, Darn!" And Thelma, laughingly said; "That's what I thought too." I was surprised to hear comments with sexual overtones from these ladies. We all laughed. They were fun to be around. They were not afraid of what people would think; they said what was on their minds. I talked often with Thelma; she was a wonderful lady who wrote beautiful poems until age of 93 when she passed away. I wasn't so sure she was appreciated as much as, I thought, she deserved. In nursing homes, this is pretty common among the elderly and their families anymore.

Their lives growing up were very different from ours and especially our children's lives. My granddaughter, Brittany, visited each evening after school. She spent quality time with these elderly ladies, made them laugh, helped them with their crafts, and at times just talked with them. It was a learning experience for her too and a blessing.

The nurses on my wing were not all familiar with some of the gadgets I had connected to me, so sometimes I would tell them how to do a procedure.

That was a switch; but, I had watched it done so many times, and my injuries were somewhat different than the routine lives of the elderly patients. It wasn't that the nurses didn't know how take care of me; they had learned the procedures throughout their training; but, they didn't work around people like me on a daily basis. I was glad when they listened to me. One lead nurse and I became pretty good friends. She came to my room at the end of her shift to change my last bandage for the day; and we would spend an hour or more talking, laughing, and learning about each others lives. She was a very interesting lady. I went home and she retired. We hadn't kept in touch except to run into each other occasionally at the Lutheran Home.

Since I was in Monroe and close for people to visit, I received even more visitors from church than when I was at Harbor Towne or Parkside. It seemed each and every one came to talk about their own set of concerns: their families, church, physical or emotional problems. I loved every minute and I learned quite a bit about listening and praying. It felt good to listen and not have to talk about things going on with me. My visitors gave me a feeling of worth. I knew everyone was curious about my condition and all the operations. I also knew the parishioners thought God had worked miracles using me and my accident. I couldn't explain to anyone my feelings, what I thought had happened, or why because it was bizarre—even to me. I needed time to digest the accident and why I survived.

On Friday mornings The Lutheran Home held church services. Wayne would attend with me. It was great! The Chaplain was so full of energy when he delivered the sermon--it was a joy to listen to him.

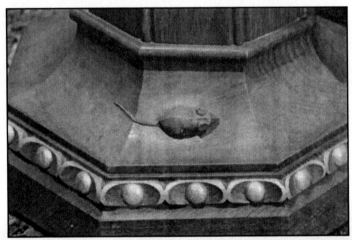

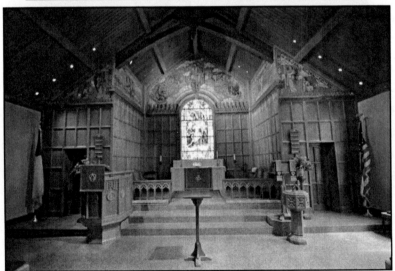

Lutheran Home Chapel

Chapter XIV

Over time Eunice and I became close friends. She was a special lady, not only to me; but, to everyone that knew her. She had lived at the nursing home for quite some time. She didn't go there to die--she made it her home. She had paintings hung on her walls--which she painted. She made crafts: sewed baby blankets, knitted and built big doll houses. She had some help with the doll houses because they were *big*. Eunice made, by hand, all of the teeny tiny furniture in the houses. She even wired one of the houses for electricity; she was an amazing woman. One of her houses was a replica of a Sears Roebuck catalogue house including the homes' actual specifications on a piece of paper.

Eunice's baby blankets were a team effort. A lady, who worked at the nursing home, would get the material squares, her companion cut the squares, Eunice would put the pattern together and sew it. While living at the nursing home, Eunice took care of some of the flowers and trees around the outside of the building. In memory of her late husband, she planted a tree outside her window with two bird houses hanging off the branches. She took a start from a lilac bush and planted it in a different location. She made sure other flowers, bushes, and trees had enough water after being planted and pulled weeds.

Eunice would ride around on a scooter with Dolly riding on the floor board at her feet--her tail hanging off the edge of the scooter. The two of them would turn heads every time they were out and about. They were so cute! On occasion Eunice would drive over Dolly's tail and pull some her hair out. Eunice would laugh and say, "Oh, poor Dolly." Dolly learned to get out of her way--most of the time. Dolly actually belonged to the Lutheran Home; but, in order for her to live there; someone had to become her caretaker. And, that someone was Eunice.

Dogs were, quite often, brought in to visit the residents. I remember once a lady brought in a beautiful Great Dane. She took the dog visiting and one elderly lady, not impressed with the dog's size, yelled, "Who let that horse in here!?" We tried to tell her the animal was a dog, but, she insisted it was a horse. Everyone standing in the hallway chuckled over the little old lady thinking the dog was a horse. Of course, it was big enough to be a pony. Dolly didn't mind sharing her home with the other animals that came to visit. I think she knew they weren't staying. Most of the time, Dolly would ignore the furry visitors, unless her Momma would pet them--that was another story.

Seven months following my entry into the Lutheran Home, it was time for doctors to take the second fixator off my left leg. Dr. Ebraheim sent me home with instructions to 'walk on it'. At this point, I had one small plate, about one and a half inches long inside my leg. The muscle flap still had an area about an inch long that would not heal and drained constantly. The leg was also still painful to put pressure on. However, since I was told to 'walk on it', that was exactly what I did. I attempted to go about my life as normally as possible; not without difficulty though. I did my best at walking normal without wobbling back and forth. I tried to distribute my weight equally on both legs. It hurt. It was a throbbing pain; but, I didn't complain. I wanted it to heal so bad I could taste it. Besides, I wasn't sure if I would ever be pain free; and, I decided I had to basically get used to the pain.

While I was home recuperating that summer, Dr. Ebraheim and the hospital opened up a new orthopedic wing at the hospital. Wayne and I had been invited to their open house. Using my walker, I walked around the new wing; and, I thought the doctor would be excited to see me up and about. However, he was more excited about his new ortho wing. I guess, I should've expected that; but, I felt a little disappointed. In my mind, my accomplishments were as great as his. In his mind, I was another routine patient. The ortho wing on the hospital was his lifetime dream, and it was a beautiful building.

Wayne decided we needed to get away from it all, so we took a weekend trip up to Frankenmuth, MI. Frankenmuth was a great little German town with all kinds of shops and hotels—a tourist attraction. The town was originally built on rolling hills. The buildings were very old and not totally handicap friendly. Wayne had to push me up the hills and hang on tight for the ride down. So much for rest and relaxation--he had quite a work out. The shops had converted their back doors for handicap access; but, finding back doors was tricky. The hotel was great; and, their hot tub was wonderful on my legs. Walking around in a bathing suit with all my scars hanging out—not a pretty sight.

Our next little jaunt that summer was to a motorcycle jamboree in Willard, Ohio. The American Legion Riders were going down there for three days and Wayne wanted me to go. It was planned I would drive the pickup and follow the motorcycles; which I thought would be okay. That was the first time I had driven any vehicle since the accident and it wasn't as easy as I figured it would be. When we got to Willard, I was a nervous wreck—to the point of tears. After getting settled into our motel, Wayne drove the pickup and left his bike parked. I was extremely happy he wanted to include me in all of the activities; but, I also felt bad. He stayed with me and didn't join in with the other riders with his bike. The trip was fun.

We met a biker called "Ice Pick", his son was "Ice Chip", and his wife was "Ice Cube". I believe they were from Texas and Ice Pick was actually a school teacher or professor. We have seen him at different jamborees and I didn't recognize him—he had a shave and a hair cut. The American Legion Riders come from all over the U.S. to attend these jamborees; and, we have met some really great people. Wayne and I came home alone and the trip went smoother, at least for me.

In August of 2007, Wayne purchased an inside booth at the Monroe County Fair to advertise the NRA, MCRGO, and his CPL classes. We spent every day at the fair attending the booth. I would sit at the booth for a while then wheel around the fair grounds talking to different people. It was wonderful to just be out and about. The fair was very tiring for us; but, it was great to be alive!

October brought about another operation. Dr. Ebraheim decided to take out my last little plate. My infectious disease doctor insisted the plate was harboring infection; and, that was the reason the muscle flap would not heal. Unhappily, I came out of the operating room with a *third* external fixator on my left leg. The bones were simply not healing. I was told the reasons for the non-union were: my age; the location of the injury; and the lack of blood flow to the area of the injury. There wasn't much to do except be patient and pray diligently.

I went home to The Lutheran Home for the second time. Praise the Lord there was room for me! This time I was at the south end of 'A' wing--last room on the right. One would have thought that location would be pretty quiet. My neighbor to the north of me arrived a day or two later. She was a very nice elderly lady; always smiling and friendly. Flora was my neighbor directly across the hall from me. She was a singer. Her favorite song was, "The Old Grey Mare Ain't What She Used to Be". The Mare was wheelchair bound and grew more and more confused as the days went by. She was the nicest little old lady until evening rolled around. Apparently, there is something called "Sundowners Syndrome". Some elderly get it when they are in their first stages of dementia. Symptoms can be irritability, confusion, anger, and acting out. The Mare had Sundowners Syndrome. She stabbed a CNA with a fork, kicked someone else, and would cuss out anyone who would try to reason with her. She was best just left alone or followed so she didn't hurt herself or anyone else.

I do believe The Mare knew God. One evening she was found in the first day room unresponsive and slumped over in her wheelchair. The nurse checked her over, ordered the CNAs to put her to bed, and observe her closely. The Mare's vitals were normal, but, it was obvious something was not quite right. Maybe an hour or two later, when the nurse checked The Mare, she found her sitting on the side of her bed: her hands and arms extended into the air over her head, her head was tilted backward, and her eyes were fixed on the ceiling. She had a big smile on her face and when the nurse walked in the door, she exclaimed, "He didn't want me, He wanted another Mare!" The nurse said The Mare's exclamation gave her chills. Did the old gray Mare see or talk to God? Only the two of them knew for sure.

Across the hall and next door to The Mare was another fine lady. She had been moved from the assisted living wing to A Wing South because her dementia had crept up on her; and, she was in need of more nursing assistance. She was able to get around on her own with the use of a walker; but, she was rough and gruff to be around. Most of the residents avoided her because her teasing was, like I said, rough and gruff. Plus, she would punch people in the arm thinking it was funny. The punchee never thought it funny; in fact, they normally got angry with her. The Puncher didn't understand why people got upset. I teased her the same way she teased me and we got along great. At night, however, she turned into a very unpleasant person. Due to being a fall risk, the Puncher was not to get up and move around her room by herself. In order to stop her from getting up and around there were alarms at her bed, chair, and the door. When one of those alarms went off, a CNA would run to assist her. Soon as her door was opened she would scream, "Close the door! Leave me alone!" If they did not leave, the Puncher was ready to fight. Once back in bed, all would be quiet for a while--another victim of 'Sundowners'. During the day, however, you could always find the Puncher sitting in the Chapel going over her rosary.

My third rowdy neighbor lived across the hall to the north of the Puncher. She was a sad case. All day, every day and into the night she would rock back and forth lamenting, "Am I going to die? When am I going to die? Are we going to die? When are we going to die? We are all going to die." The nurses and CNAs tried very hard to talk with her in an attempt to calm her down— to no avail. When Wayne visited, the constant lamenting got to him. She was so mournful. The Mare would yell at her, "Yes, we going to die! So, be quiet!" Then The Mare would grumble something under her breath, shake her head, and mosey off. That interaction between the two of them was comical in a sorrowful sort of way. Just when I thought they were in their own little worlds and not paying any attention to anyone else; The Mare would get irritated and answer Lamentation.

The CNAs thought Lamentation was afraid of dying. They thought she didn't know Jesus, because her every waking hour was asking about death. It was very sad. My husband thought Lamentation was not healthy for me to be around. He thought her woeful chanting would depress me; so, he asked if I could be moved to another room. Wayne was also worried about my lack of rest. All three of my noisy neighbors contributed to my lack of rest; however, my next door neighbor was a gem.

I was moved to another room on 'A' wing north, one room away from Eunice and Dolly. Perfect! The 'Sunshine Girl' was in between us. Sunny was usually a quiet lady, except, if she had to go to the bathroom. Sunny wasn't supposed to get out of her wheelchair by herself and there was an alarm on the bathroom door. She would open the door, the alarm would go off, and so did she. Sunny would *slam* the door shut grumbling loudly all the time because the noise was so loud. She didn't need a call button; she could be heard all the way down the hall cussing at the door alarm.

My granddaughter, Brittany, came to the Lutheran Home after school until her mother picked her up after work. Sunny and Brittany would play in Sunny's room. You could hear Sunny laughing up a storm at Brittany. I would check in on them to see what was going on and Sunny would say, "She's alright, we're just playing."

When Sunny passed, a Hospice volunteer was sitting with her late at night in her room. I could hear the volunteer, tearfully, tell Sunny it was okay to let go. It was okay to go live with Jesus. I wondered if Sunny knew what the Hospice lady was telling her—Sunny passed that night. It was a blessing.

The next lady who moved into Sunny's room was quite a character. She was almost 99 years old, outspoken, and at times down right mean. No body could do anything right according to her-- not the staff and not her family. She was a very unhappy woman. Her actions and language was awful. Her son had to have a talk with. He advised her that if she didn't straighten up, he didn't know what they were going to do with her. She had been in a few other nursing homes and didn't like them either. Her children were at the end of the road with her. Once Grumpy's son rebuked her for bad behavior, she calmed down--some. She had a scowl on her face most of the time and talking to her was near impossible. Her adult children visited every day like clock work. Grumpy used one of her daughters as a whipping post. Every visit she vented on that lady—to the point of running her away. The daughter would leave, return another day, and Grumpy would start all over again.

One day a CNA was in Grumpy's room helping her when, all of a sudden, I heard the CNA calling for help. The CNAs partner was in another room with a patient and couldn't hear the CNAs calls. I turned my call light on, wheeled through the bathroom into Grumpy's room., coming up behind her. The CNA was standing over Grumpy--almost in tears. Grumpy was biting down on the CNAs arm. I put my fingers on Grumpy's jaw bones and pressed; as if I was trying to get an animal to let go of whatever it was holding in its mouth. I was talking to Grumpy too--attempting to convince her to open her mouth. By the time the second CNA got to the room, Grumpy had let go of the first CNAs arm. Poor thing had deep teeth marks in her arm; but, the skin wasn't broken. The lesson--don't put your arm in front of an old lady's face. False teeth or not the bite will hurt.

During those three months at the Lutheran Home, I managed to go with Eunice to Thursday evening Bible study. Eunice still wouldn't play bingo; but, we sure had a good time after bingo--drinking our coffee, eating our snacks, and talking. In the evenings, I spent a lot of time in Eunice's room conversing with her about everything and anything. She showed me her picture albums that held all of her life's memories: her home, antiques, and her family; which she was very proud of. She tried to show me how to knit socks. I watched her intently trying to figure out the pattern--never did understand it. She made at least four pair of socks and she wore them too.

Eunice taught me the difference between a dish rag and a dish cloth. She made dish cloths--not dish rags. She also told me that dinner was served at noon and supper served at night. In my world, it was breakfast, lunch, and dinner. Not at the Lutheran Home; it was breakfast, dinner, and supper. My elder was teaching me etiquette. Eunice had many visitors every day. She was a wonderful person to visit with. She was definitely a Christian with spunk.

While I was laid up, I decided to go back to school and work for a Paralegal Certificate. The courses were accelerated seven week courses; but, all I had was time. Wayne brought my laptop, to me, and the home let me get on their internet. I was all set to study. I spent a lot of time working on my lessons, in therapy, running to the doctor, playing bingo, and spending time with Eunice.

Dolly spent a lot of time in my room. I would be in Eunice's room visiting with her and Dolly would get up, walk out of the room, trot down the hall, and into my room. I would watch her. She would stop in the doorway, turn around and look back at me as if saying, "Come on, I want a treat!" I would go back to my room, get her a treat; which she would eat, and trot right back to Eunice's room. Dolly had her work cut out for her keeping an eye on both me and Eunice. Dolly made my days. I was having a hard time staying upbeat. It's been three and a half years and I was still living in a nursing home waiting for my bones to heal. Waking up to Dolly grunting at me because she wanted a treat was the best.

Eunice contracted the flu and was sick for about a week. I became very worried about her. Eunice's daughter, Mary, was a cancer survivor and her immune system was weak so she would call Eunice instead of visit. I wanted to see her so I went to her room, knocked on the door, and went inside. Eunice told me not to stay she was afraid I would get sick. I told her not to worry; I had many antibiotics in my system. On her table was a full tray of food; which Eunice did not feel like eating. Instead of that regular meal, I asked a CNA to get her some soup. Then I sat by her bedside and read aloud to her the Portals of Prayer, the Bible verses and a prayer. When the soup arrived, I left so the CNA could help her eat. In a couple days Eunice was up, around, and back to being herself. Thank you, Lord. That spunky little lady and her puppy dog meant the world to me.

So far, the reports and x-rays of my leg looked pretty good. Dr. Ebraheim was confident the last bone graph would work; as long as I didn't do something stupid. Believe me; I worked very hard to get back on my feet. At this point, I felt virtually pain free. At times, I would put a little weight on my foot and fixator to test it--no pain.

Thanksgiving, 2010, and I was spending it at the Lutheran Home--for the second year. The Lutheran Home did a real nice job with their Thanksgiving dinners. That year Wayne's Aunt Claribel had come to live in the nursing home too; so, we would be eating together on A Wing porch. It seemed strange having a relative in the nursing home with me. Claribel lived in the assisted living wing at the other end of the building; but, I saw her everyday. I was glad she was there. We had been very worried about her living alone. She told me she had fallen twice at her apartment. She hadn't gotten hurt; but, she didn't want my mother-in-law to know about her falls. I advised her to think about putting her name on the active admissions list at the Lutheran Home--which she did.

Claribel had issues with clogged arteries and her condition required stints to be inserted; however, one artery was too plugged to receive a stint. She was too fragile and the artery could not be opened. She was pretty thin and shaky; and, her heart was not pumping at full strength. Someone at the nursing home would be watching her at all times; which was a relief to the family was. She was in therapy to keep up her strength and keep her moving. We could see that her health was going down hill. Her spirits were up; but, her body was not willing.

One afternoon, while Wayne and I were peacefully sitting in my room watching TV, a tall, older man with graying hair came to my door. He looked inside my room and said, "Hello" to Wayne; then said he had come to visit me. He introduced himself to us, and asked Wayne if he remembered him—he had worked with Wayne's Dad many years prior. This man told us, the reason he had come to talk with me was--he had been at my accident. He said he had been following my progress via a friend from our church. He heard I was back at the Lutheran Home, and, decided it was time to pay me a visit. Wayne and I looked at each other in amazement. He began to tell us his version of my accident--which was quite different from any version we had heard thus far.

This man's unexpected recollection of the accident went like this--he was a motorcycle rider and rode Albain Road every day. He said he came up to the accident seconds after it had happened. He rode past Wayne, who was running back to me and, at the same time, was on his cell phone calling for help. The man claimed, he pulled up ahead of all the vehicles involved, stopped, and walked back to the accident to see if he could help. He said, he heard me gurgling as I tried to breathe. He thought the motorcycle was on top of me; and, he could see my feet sticking out from under the bike. He said he heard people discussing moving the bike off of me; which, he didn't think would be a good idea. He picked my helmet up and set it off to the side of the road. Then he decided he couldn't do anything so he left. He rode home, told his wife about the accident, and the two of them returned to the scene. By the time they returned, I was gone; but, the vehicles and officers were still on scene. He talked to an officer for a few minutes, and told him what he witnessed. He said every time he rides around that curve; he's reminded of that day--what he saw and heard. Since the accident, he had been tracking my progress. It had been three years, and he was happy to finally talk to me. I gave him a hug, thanked him for his concern, prayers, and visit. After that man left, Wayne and I sat in silence for quite a while. His description of the accident aroused questions in my mind. He had said things I hadn't heard before, and Wayne looked puzzled.

Sometime in November I went back to the doctor, and he was ready to take off my fixator. He was anxious to get me up walking. I had talked with people who had taken off their own fixators, so I asked him if I could take mine off in the office. He smiled at me and said, "Sure, if you want to." I looked at him and asked, "Will it hurt?" He said, "We'll do it in surgery." Guess that answered my question. They set me up for my last surgery, number (42), December 10, 2010. Following that fixator removal, I was fitted for a brace to wear on my foot and leg. I ordered a pair of shoes--extra wide on the left side. Plus, they had to be raised one inch on the left side. The right side was my regular size and width. I was told to buy two pair of shoes—different sizes.

The leg brace arrived and December 23, 2010—same day I went home. That was the best Christmas ever; no decorations, no family get together; just home *to stay*. At least once a week, I returned to the nursing home to visit Eunice and Dolly. Sometimes we would go to the dining room for coffee or I brought two coffees to her room. On the last Friday of the month, we would go to Chapel for communion. I would help take residents to the Chapel service and back to their rooms. On some visits, I would give Dolly baths. Eunice thought the home was a little slack on her grooming so I tried to help out. Dolly would get pretty excited when she saw me coming down the hall. Her tail wagged and her body wiggled all over.

Chapter XV

Eventually, Eunice gave in and started playing bingo; which surprised me, because, I thought she didn't like it. Oh well, she was cute. Wayne volunteered the American Legion and AM Vets to do bingo at the Lutheran Home on the third Monday of each month. One of the American Legion gentlemen called it for them until his wife passed away. Then I took over for him. The rest of our volunteers handed out the prizes or helped the ladies find their numbers and their bingos. The ladies at the nursing home looked forward to us coming in each month. The prizes were donated by our church which was great. I had a wonderful time visiting with the ladies and calling bingo.

One afternoon, Wayne and I were out and about shopping; and, I went into the store's bathroom. I stood up from the toilet, turned to flush; and, I felt a sharp shooting pain go up my left leg. My reaction was, *"Oh, S__t! That hurt!"* Then I thought, *"Maybe I really didn't do what I think I just did."* The shopping cart was outside the door, and, due to the pain, I hobbled to it. I found Wayne and told him we had to leave. I advised him I had done something to my leg and it wasn't good. I hoped the weather might have been the cause of my pain; because, my leg was aching before we went into the store.

I tried to ignore the pain—it would not go away. Wayne wanted to stop at a restaurant for dinner. He wanted to ask for a gift certificate to give away at an NRA dinner planned for September.

Anyway, I managed to get through our dinner and get home. I put my therapeutic boot on; which helped a little with the pain. I accidently stepped down hard with my left leg which caused even more pain. I went to the couch and sat down. Wayne asked if I wanted to go to the hospital. I wanted to give my leg time--hoping the pain would go away. I told Wayne to go to his gun club meeting; and, if I needed him, I would call. He said he would be home early.

In the meantime, my daughter and her friend stopped by to visit. We talked for a little while, and then Aprell's friend went for hamburgers. When he returned, we went into the kitchen to eat. My leg was hurting so badly, I could barely get to the table. Aprell called Wayne to come home and take me to the hospital; which he did.

As we drove to the hospital, every bump shot pain up my leg. In the emergency room, the pain was so intense, I could not move without screaming. X-rays were taken, and sure enough, I cracked the bone again! I was given pain medicine and told to come back in two weeks when I was already scheduled to see the doctor. When I went to see Dr. Ebraheim, he walked into the room and said, "I know, you broke it again." "I'll fix it." He was *not* happy with me.

Following more x-rays, the Doctor put me in a walking cast and told me to return in four weeks. Four weeks later the cast was replaced with another cast. This second cast rubbed the front of my leg and created a half dollar sized blister. That cast was removed after a week. Instead of replacing the cast for a third time, they put me back in a therapeutic boot--my second. The boot made it easy for me to access the blister to keep it medicated and clean.

Wayne took me to a Republican Reagan Day Dinner sometime in the fall--my second dinner. The first one I went to from the Lutheran Home; and, in a wheelchair. The next one I went to from home with a boot and a walker. While outside waiting for Wayne to bring the car around, I was talking to a pastor's wife who said; "I bet you never thought you would be walking like this, did you?" I have to admit she took me by surprise with her comment and I looked at her and replied; "I never thought I wouldn't." She said, "You probably never realized how bad you were like the rest of us did." She was right and praise the Lord I didn't have negative thoughts.

I, also, went to a church meeting where I met my brother-in-law's step-daughter. She was the lady who held me at the accident scene until the helicopter arrived. We got to talking and she gave me her version of the accident. I had wanted to talk to her for quite some time. I wanted to hear her version of what happened at the scene. She told me she had been at a house party for Memorial Day when she heard the crash. Two men from the house went to find out what had happened. Upon returning to the house, they stated to my step-niece and a nurse that they probably should go to the scene to help with the injured person--me. My niece said when she came running up on me, she thought I was a child—I was lying in a bunch. She sat down in the road; put my head in between her legs to keep me from moving. At first, I was unconscious. A short time later, I regained consciousness. I was talking normal. I wanted to get up. I couldn't figure out why I was on the ground. My niece, of course, would not let me get up. I couldn't anyway. My bones were all broke and I was bleeding internally. She talked to me and argued with Wayne; who thought my helmet should be removed. She wouldn't let him do that. The motorcycle was next to me and it was leaking gas; so, a couple of guys moved the bike away from me. The nurse on scene desperately tried to convince the Life-Flite helicopter to fly to the scene. However, her call was prior to the EMTS arriving.

The two women were trying to keep me from going into shock. The nurse did not think I would survive if the helicopter didn't get me to a hospital as soon as possible. After the EMTS arrived, the fire chief radioed the helicopter and he convinced them to immediately detour to my location. My brother-in-law arrived on the scene; and, at that time, my step-niece realized who Wayne and I were. Until then, she said we looked familiar, but wasn't sure exactly who we were.

Interestingly, the motorcycle had not landed on top of me; but, beside me. The man, who worked with Wayne's Dad, must have thought the bike was lying on me from the angle he observed the scene. I did not have chest injuries; but, I was bleeding inside. I commented earlier, about the different versions of what witnesses thought they saw at the accident scene. Each individual saw things from a different perspective. I was glad I was able to talk with my step-niece and heard her version. It was interesting to me. I wanted to know everything about it. I hoped my memory would eventually return. Nothing seemed to be jogging those brain cells.

For six more weeks I walked around in the boot before returning to the doctor's clinic. My x-rays looked good. The bone graph is building bone and filling in between the fibula and tibia nicely. Doctor was pleased. He gave me three months between appointments. Praise God!

I had been home for about six months; and, except for the bone cracking when I went to the bathroom at the store, all seemed well. By the way, when I cracked the bone, the interns at the hospital kept saying 'I fell'. I did not fall; I twisted my legs when I turned to flush the toilet. My legs did not turn with my body. I twisted and the bone cracked.

Summer, 2010, Wayne bought a Harley Davidson with a wrap around seat for me to ride in. My first time back on the bike was exciting. Wayne on the other hand was a nervous wreck. I think he anticipated what my reactions might to be when we got on the road. I was fine We took a couple of test runs to make sure I wasn't going to panic or freak out--I didn't. I don't remember the accident at all. Consequently, I wasn't afraid. Besides, I wanted to live life not being afraid of what might happen. I believed God and His angels were with us; and, He has a plan for each of us.

July 4th weekend, 2010, my daughter and I drove out to the State of Washington. She rented a van, packed her things in it and we drove from Monroe, Michigan to Kalama, Washington. Aprell was going to live with her biological Dad and step-mother--with my blessing. The trip took about a week for us to drive. Aprell saw landscape she had never seen before; and, it brought back childhood memories for me. We laughed like we haven't laughed before. It was a great trip for the two of us.

I dropped Aprell off in Kalama, and then I drove to Seattle, Washington--about three hours north. I flew home out of Sea-Tac Airport into Detroit Metro. Wayne was supposed to meet me at the airport; but, we didn't set up a meeting area. It was a blessing we found each other. I was walking down the corridor sort of in a daze. I was so tired. I looked up, and there was Wayne coming down the escalator. Praise God! I was so glad and relieved; because, I didn't know the first place to look for him. The airport was so big. He got me a wheelchair; my legs were aching and tired. I had tripped a couple of times and caught myself. I was glad to be home.

People said they were surprised at me; and, hadn't expected me to do some of the things I did after having gone through so much. No one expected me to get back on a motorcycle, drive 2000 miles with my daughter, and flying back by myself. I didn't find those things unusual. Often, I had been told that I was a tough old lady. I don't consider myself tough, stubborn maybe, not tough. Not afraid—as long as God was with me.

Eunice was one of the people worried about me. She was concerned about my going on such a long trip so soon after getting home from the nursing home and hospitals. I knew I was in her prayers. I visited and gave Dolly a bath as soon as I returned home. I told her all about the trip and showed her the pictures. Her and Dolly were happy to see me; which made me feel good.

Next, Wayne and I took a motorcycle trip to Milwaukee, Wisconsin with the American Legion Riders. We rode to Muskegon, Michigan, took the jet ferry over to Milwaukee, and joined other riders for the yearly jamboree. It was a hot ride, but a good ride. We enjoyed ourselves. We visited the Harley Davidson Museum and the Milwaukee Brewery. Plus there were merchandising booths set up at the expo building, a dinner one night, presentations and raffles. A good time was had by all.

In September, Wayne and I had been asked to help with the Lutheran Home's yearly Country Fair. I walked in the front door expecting to see Eunice. As I walked up on her open door, I thought something was not quite right. Eunice was lying in her bed—sleeping. It was very unusual for her to sleep with her door open. She looked so frail and pitiful. My heart sank. A week prior, I had been to visit with her and she was doing well. In fact, it was funny. Wayne dropped me off at the home to visit with Eunice for the afternoon. It was getting late, and I had begun to wonder where Wayne was. Eunice and I were talking about that very thing, when Wayne popped in the door and said, "I got almost home and realized I forgot to pick Sandy up." Eunice and I burst into loud laughter. He forgot me! Eunice thought that was the funniest she had heard in a long time. And, I loved her laughter. So, what happened after that visit?

I asked the nurse, who told me to let her rest. He said she had many visitors that day and she was tired. I complied, and went to the dining room. I ran into a lady who said it was thought Eunice had a heart attack. At that point, I didn't care what the nurse thought; I wanted to sit by Eunice's side for a little while. I left Wayne visiting with other people, and I went back to Eunice's room. I thought I could take Dolly outside or something. Wayne didn't stay in the dining room—he followed me. He took Dolly outside, she wouldn't go with me. When she heard Wayne's voice she took off to the doors. We tried to be quiet; but, Eunice woke up. She didn't say too much except, "Hello". She did know us; and, thanked Wayne for taking care of Dolly. I read her the Daily Devotion for the day, then she drifted off to sleep and we left.

I felt so sad; my best friend was dying. For the next three weeks, I called the Lutheran Home daily or stopped in to sit with her. I would read the daily devotions to her. She knew me every time I visited. Her mind was good. She said, "You know, I'm ready, don't you." I said, "I do know that; but, I'm not ready to let you go." She smiled and nodded. At another visit, I came into Eunice's room and she was sleeping. I quietly got a chair to sit next to her bed, when she woke up and started crying. She held her arm out to me and exclaimed, "Oh, Sandy!" By the way she sounded, I thought she was in pain; but, when I asked she said, "No, I'm just so glad to see you." I knelt down by the side of the bed and held her in my arms. I said to her, "We had some really good times here, didn't we." She chuckled and said, "Yes, we did. And, I'm looking forward to seeing you and Wayne again someday." I replied, "Me too, I love you."

The CNAs kept a chart on Dolly as well as Eunice. They were keeping track of when she went outside and when she ate. It was cute and, I thought, quite appropriate.

One afternoon, I ran into Eunice's daughter, Mary, at the grocery store. She was getting Eunice some key lime pie. We started talking and she told me Eunice's problem wasn't a heart attack. Her cancer from years ago had returned. They had found two tumors--one in her lung and one in her liver. She wasn't in any pain. Mary told me a cute story about Eunice. The Lutheran

Home social worker asked her mom if she ever had a drinking problem. Eunice laughed and said, "Just my husband." (Eunice's husband had been an alcoholic for many years prior to his passing.) Even in death, Eunice still had her wit and humor. September 28, 2011 Eunice passed away. The Lutheran Home had Dolly put to sleep, as well. Dolly couldn't have lived with anyone else. She couldn't hear, she had cataracts, her teeth were falling out, and she was losing control of her body functions. Dolly knew what was going on with Eunice; you could see it in the way she acted.

The funeral was held at the Lutheran Home. When I walked in, I saw Mary right away. She advised me where the casket was sitting inside the chapel; and, that Dolly was in the casket with Eunice. I was stunned! I must have looked stunned too. Mary explained, Dolly had been put to sleep—her remains cremated. Dolly's ashes were in a velveteen bag next to Eunice in the casket. I was relieved--Eunice and Dolly were together. I turned and told Wayne that Dolly was in the casket with Eunice. He looked as shocked as I had been. I could hear Eunice's laughter at the look on his face. I smiled, shook my head, and said, "Come here I'll show you." We entered the chapel; which was full of Eunice's friends and relatives. Eunice looked so pretty and natural--the velvet bag was lying by her side.

The chaplain told many great things about Eunice and her sense of humor. Recently, he had been in a motorcycle accident had to have surgery on his nose. After a doctor's checkup, he went to visit with Eunice The first comment he made to her was, "Boy, I've had quite a day." Eunice smiled and replied, "Tell me about it." He knew immediately what he had said, he smiled to himself and said, "I guess, I don't have to tell you what kind of a day I had". He said he couldn't talk about Eunice without talking about Dolly. The two were like 'peas in a pod'. Wherever Eunice would be, Dolly wasn't far away. Eunice and Dolly looked after each other as if they were family. The two of them passing at the same time, was a blessing.

Eunice's funeral was the hardest one we had been to in years. Wayne's eyes swelled up with tears and I sobbed uncontrollably. Someone asked me if I would return to the Lutheran Home with Eunice and Dolly gone. I had no intensions not to return. I still had friends there, and I loved visiting the home. A beautiful picture of Eunice and Dolly; along with a plaster cast of

Dolly's footprint were placed in a glass wall case at the Lutheran Home. A big picture of Eunice with me behind her was hung in the front door hall. Eunice and Dolly are now a part of the Lutheran Home's history. Tuesday, February 21st, Eunice would have been 90 years young. I was so blessed to have been a minuscule part of her life. The two of them will be in my heart forever.

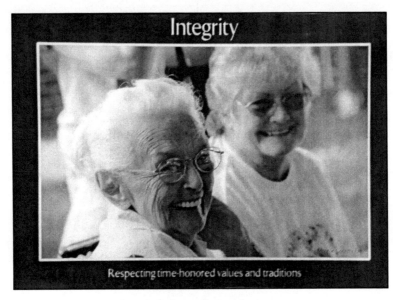

Eunice & Sandy

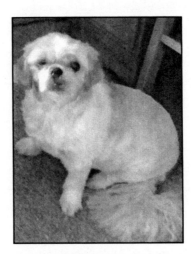

Dolly (puppy dog)

In December, 2011, I went to the doctor for another checkup. After the x-rays were looked at, Dr. Ebraheim exclaimed; "It looks good, it's a 'miracle', it looks really good." The bone graph was doing its job--making more bone and connecting the two bones together. Best of all, I don't have to return for another check up for a year. If I could have jumped up and down in excitement, I would have. I have had ongoing problems with getting lightheaded, dizzy, and balance. I definitely do not have any complaints. God truly worked many 'Miracles' through me and Wayne. I love Him and I praise Him.

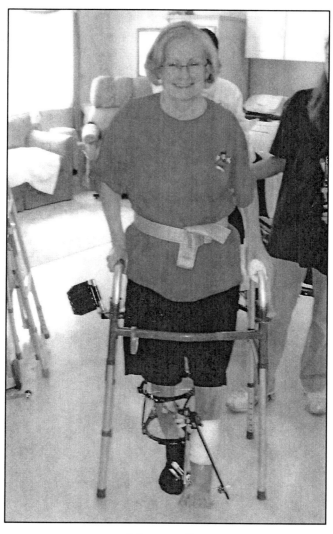

Me on walker

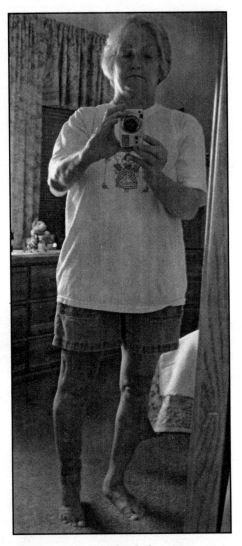

Me healed.

A long time ago, I read a poem that, at the time, I thought was pretty cute. I thought to myself, I would have liked to have been known for the type of person the poem was talking about. However, I hadn't lived the type of lifestyle that would have fulfilled my thoughts. Motorcycle riding hadn't been part of my life. I looked at my scarred, and broken body, and I thought--I'm not so sure. The poem is: "Life's Journey" written by Mavis Leyrer, age 83 from Seattle, Washington; and it goes like this:

Life's journey is not to arrive safely at the grave

In a well preserved body

But rather to skid in sideways totally worn out shouting

Holy S__t...What a Ride!

No, to my knowledge, Ms. Leyrer, was not a motorcycle rider; but, I was. If I had not taken up riding a motorcycle, I would've missed part of my 'Life's Journey'. Praise God!

The End

Bible Verses

From

New International Version Bible

[24] A person's steps are directed by the LORD. How then can anyone understand their own way?

[5] Trust in the LORD with all your heart and lean not on your own understanding

[28] And we know that in all things God works for the good of those who love him, who[a] have been called according to his purpose.

[38] For I am convinced that neither death nor life, neither angels nor demons,[a] neither the present nor the future, nor any powers,

[39] neither height nor depth, nor anything else in all creation, will be able to separate us from the love of God that is in Christ Jesus our Lord.

Romans 15:13............................[13] May the God of hope fill you with all joy and peace as you trust in him, so that you may overflow with hope by the power of the Holy Spirit.

Philippians 4:6............................[6] Do not be anxious about anything, but in every situation, by prayer and petition, with thanksgiving, present your requests to God.

Jeremiah 9:8............................[8] Their tongue is a deadly arrow; it speaks deceitfully. With their mouths they all speak cordially to their neighbors, but in their hearts they set traps for them.

Romans 2:21............................[21] you, then, who teach others, do you not teach yourself? You who preach against stealing, do you steal?

Jeremiah 17:14............................[14] Heal me, LORD, and I will be healed; save me and I will be saved, for you are the one I praise.

Jeremiah 29:11............................[11] For I know the plans I have for you," declares the LORD, "plans to prosper you and not to harm you, plans to give you hope and a future.

Genesis 2:21.............................[21] So the LORD God caused the man to fall into a deep sleep;

1 Samuel 26:12..........................[12] So David took the spear and water jug near Saul's head, and they left. No one saw or knew about it, nor did anyone wake up. They were all sleeping, because the LORD had put them into a deep sleep.

Acts 14:22.................................[22] strengthening the disciples and encouraging them to remain true to the faith. "We must go through many hardships to enter the kingdom of God," they said.

Galatians 3:5.............................[5] So again I ask, does God give you his Spirit and work miracles among you by the works of the law, or by your believing what you heard?

Matthew 26:39..........................[39] Going a little farther, he fell with his face to the ground and prayed, "My Father, if it is possible, may this cup be taken from me. Yet not as I will, but as you will.

Psalms 20:1..............................[1] May the LORD answer you when you are in distress; may the name of the God of Jacob protect you.

Psalms 46:1..............................[1] God is our refuge and strength, an ever-present help in trouble

Psalms 91:11............................[11] For he will command his angels concerning you to guard you in all your ways;

Joshua 1:9...................................[9] Have I not commanded you? Be strong and courageous. Do not be afraid; do not be discouraged, for the LORD your God will be with you wherever you go."

1 Corinthians 3:15.....................[15] But in your hearts revere Christ as Lord. Always be prepared to give an answer to everyone who asks you to give the reason for the hope that you have. But do this with gentleness and respect,

1 Peter 5:7..............................[7] Cast all your anxiety on him because he cares for you.

Ephesians 2:5 & 8......................[5] Cast all your anxiety on him because he cares for you. [8]For it is **by grace** you have been **saved**, through faith—and this is not from yourselves, it is the gift of **God.**